THE EIGHT PIECES OF BROCADE
Improving and Maintaining Health

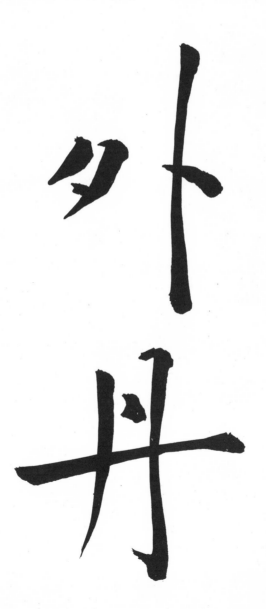

BY DR. YANG JWING-MING

DISCLAIMER

The author(s) and publisher of this material are **NOT RESPONSI-BLE** in any manner whatsoever for any injury which may occur through reading or following the instructions in this material.

The activities, physical and otherwise, described in this material may be too strenuous or dangerous for some people, and the reader(s) should consult a physician before engaging in them.

© YANG'S MARTIAL ARTS ASSOCIATION (YMAA), 1988, 1992

10, 10

All right reserved

ISBN: 0-940871-05-X

Library of Congress No: 88-050012

Publisher's Cataloging in Publication
(Prepared by Quality Books Inc.)

Yang, Jwing-Ming, 1946-
    The eight pieces of brocade : a wai dan chi kung exercise set / by
Yang Jwing-Ming. -- 2nd ed.
    (YMAA book series ; 10)
    Chinese and English.
    ISBN 0-940871-05-X

   1. Ch'i kung. 2. T'ai chi ch'uan. 3. Exercise.   I. Title. II.
Title: A wai dan chi kung exercise set. III. Series.

   RA781.8   613.7'148
                                        88-50012

Distrubuted by the Talman Company

Printed in Hong Kong

YMAA PUBLICATION CENTER
YANG'S MARTIAL ARTS ASSOCIATION (YMAA)
38 HYDE PARK AVENUE
JAMAICA PLAIN, MASSACHUSETTS 02130

ACKNOWLEDGEMENT

Thanks to A. Reza Farman-Farmaian for the photography, David Ripianzi, David Dollars, Eric Hoffman, and James O'Leary, Jr. for proofing the manuscript and contributing many valuable suggestions and discussions, and Christer Manning and Douglas Goodman for the drawings and cover design. Special thanks to Alan Dougall for his editing.

ABOUT THE AUTHOR
DR. YANG JWING-MING

Dr. Yang was born in Taiwan, Republic of China, in 1946. He started his Kung Fu/Wushu training at the age of fifteen under the Shaolin White Crane (Pai Huo) master Cheng Gin-Gsao. At sixteen Dr. Yang began the study of Tai Chi Chuan (Yang Style) under Master Kao Tao.

Dr. Yang practiced Tai Chi with Master Kao for nearly three years. During this period, he learned the Yang style barehand form, Tai Chi breathing, and Chi circulation exercises. This was the beginning of Dr. Yang's involvement with Chi Kung. Through his Tai Chi practice, Dr. Yang gained an understanding of the fundamentals of Chi Kung training, especially the sitting practice for small circulation (Shao Jou Tian).

When Dr. Yang was eighteen, he entered Tamkang College in Taipei Hsien to study Physics. While there, he began the study of Shaolin Long Fist (Chang Chuan) with Master Li Mao-Ching. At the same time, he advanced his Tai Chi training with Master Li. Later, he also practiced and studied together with his classmate Mr. Wilson Chen, who was learning Tai Chi Chuan with one of the most famous Tai Chi masters in Taipei, Master Chang Shyang-Shan. From these efforts, and through the continued studying of Tai Chi and Chi Kung books, Dr. Yang and Mr. Chen were able to greatly increase their understanding of the internal arts.

In 1971 Dr. Yang completed his M.S. degree in Physics at the National Taiwan University, and then served in the Chinese Air Force. After discharge, he returned to Tamkang College to teach Physics and resume study under Master Li Mao-Ching.

In 1974, Dr. Yang came to the United States to study Mechanical Engineering at Purdue University. Dr. Yang founded the Purdue University Chinese Kung Fu Research Club and also taught college credited courses in Tai Chi Chuan. In 1978 he was awarded a Ph.D. in Mechanical Engineering.

In 1980, Dr. Yang went to Houston and worked for Texas Instruments. While in Houston he founded Yang's Shaolin Kung Fu Academy, which was taken over by his student, Mr. Jeffery Bolt, after he moved to Boston in 1982. While Dr. Yang was continuing his engineering career, he also founded Yang's Martial Arts Academy (YMAA) on October 1, 1982 in Boston.

In 1984 he resigned his engineering job so that he could concentrate his efforts on teaching and writing about the Chinese martial arts and Chi Kung. Dr. Yang has been deeply involved in studying and researching Chi Kung, and has shared his knowledge through numerous lectures and seminars. Dr. Yang has written ten books on these subjects, and has published five videotapes.

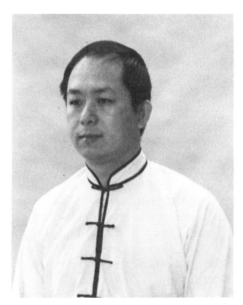

Dr. Yang, Jwing-Ming

FOREWORD

Since Chinese acupuncture was introduced to the Western world, the idea of Chi and its circulation in the human body has gradually become recognized and accepted by Western doctors and the general public. More and more people in this country are turning to acupuncture treatments or trying Chi Kung, and as they tell their friends of their good experiences, the reputation of these Oriental arts increases.

Practicing Chi Kung (which is working with Chi, the energy within the body) can not only maintain your health and mental balance, but can also cure a number of illnesses without the use of any drugs. Chi Kung uses either still or moving meditation to increase and regulate the Chi circulation.

When you practice regularly, your mind will gradually become calm and peaceful, and your whole being will start to feel more balanced. However, the most important thing that will come from the regular practice of Chi Kung is your discovery of the inner world of your body's energy. Through sensing and feeling, and examining your inner experiences, you will start to understand yourself not only physically but also mentally. This science of internal sensing, which the Chinese have been studying for several thousand years, is usually totally ignored by the Western world. However, in today's busy and confusing society, this training is especially important. With the mental peace and calmness that Chi Kung can give you, you will be better able to relax and enjoy your daily work, and perhaps even find real happiness.

I believe that it is very important for the Western world to learn, study, research, and develop this scientific internal art on a wide scale immediately. I sincerely believe that it can be very effective in helping people, especially young people, to cope with the confusing and frightening challenges of life. The general practice of Chi Kung would reduce the mental pressure in our society, help those who are unbalanced, and perhaps even lower the crime rate. Chi Kung balances the internal energy and can heal many illnesses. Older people especially will find that it will maintain their health and even slow the aging process. In addition, Chi Kung will help older people to conquer depression and worry, and to find peace, calm, and real happiness. I am confident that people in the Western world will realize, as have millions of Chinese, that Chi Kung practice will give them a new outlook on life, and that it will turn out to be a key to solving many of today's problems.

For these reasons, I have been actively studying, researching, and publishing what I have learned. However, after a few years of effort, I feel that what I have accomplished is too slow and shallow. The reason for this is simply that YMAA is young and lacks the financial foundation to handle such a large and important job. I and the few people like me who are struggling to spread the word about Chi Kung cannot do it well enough by ourselves. We need to get more people involved, but we especially need to have universities and established medical organizations get involved in the research.

YMAA has established a department for Chi Kung study and research. We will continue working to introduce this knowledge to the public through seminars, books, and videotapes. The only thing keeping us from researching deeper and more quickly is our limited financial foundation.

To conclude, I would like to point out one thing to those of you who are sincerely interested in studying and researching this "new" science. If you start now, future generations will view you as a pioneer of the scientific investigation of Chi Kung. In addition to improving your own health, you will share the credit for raising our understanding of life as well as increasing the store of happiness in this world.

PREFACE

Since my first Chi Kung book, "Chi Kung Health and Martial Arts", was published, I have received countless letters and phone calls. Almost all of them are to express people's gratitude for the benefit they have received from practicing the Chi Kung exercises introduced in the book. Surprisingly, many of the readers are Western doctors who have been applying Chi Kung theory and teaching the exercises to their patients — and obtaining very positive results. Many of them have suggested that I produce videotapes to help people learn the exercises more accurately and efficiently.

With this encouragement, I have been studying and researching more deeply, trying to increase my understanding of the exercises. After three years of study and practice, I have decided to publish these videotapes. The first tape will introduce one of the most common and basic Chi Kung exercises in China — The Eight Pieces of Brocade. This set of exercises was created by Marshal Yeuh Fei during the Southern Sung dynasty (1127-1279 A.D.) for improving his soldiers' health. Since that time, these exercises have become one of the most popular exercises in China.

There are a number of reasons for introducing this set first: 1. Its theory and training methods are the simplest and easiest to understand. It is therefore the best set for the Chi Kung beginner. 2. If you practice this set regularly, you should be able to notice improvements in your health within a few months. 3. The set can be practiced by anybody, young or old, healthy or sick. 4. This set will give you a good understanding of basic Chi Kung theory, so that if you wish, you may go on to more advanced training.

Although it is best to use this manual together with the videotape, it is possible to learn the set using this manual alone. Seeing the set done will clear up many small questions, and avoid the ambiguities inherent in any printed description or still photograph. However, if you read carefully and proceed step by step, you should be able to grasp the essentials well enough to gain full benefit from the exercises.

If there proves to be enough of a demand for manuals and videotapes such as these, YMAA will publish a continuing series of Chi Kung training materials. These materials will introduce a number of different Chi Kung sets and explain the theoretical background for each. At present, a series of ten videotapes and manuals is envisioned, ranging from basic to advanced.

In addition, I am working on a series of books which will discuss in greater depth the various styles of Chi Kung. The first book will lay down the theoretical foundation, or root, of Chi Kung. This will give you a general understanding of the theory and principles, which is necessary if you wish to further your study. The second book in this series will be on

Marrow Washing Chi Kung. Marrow Washing Chi Kung has been known in China (although it has been kept secret) since the Liang dynasty, more than fourteen hundred years ago. Marrow washing is deep, and difficult to understand, but once mastered it can give you the health of a child, increase your resistance to disease, and even lengthen your life.

The third volume will be concerned with Chi Kung cavity press healing. It will help people understand the basic principles of acupressure. Cavity press Chi Kung healing is the root of Japanese Shiatsu Massage. The fourth volume will cover Chi Kung and health, including basic principles as well as various styles of Chi Kung designed to improve the health or to treat specific ailments. The next volume will concern Chi Kung training that the martial artist can use to improve his fighting potential, such as Shaolin Chi Kung training methods, iron shirt, and iron sand palm. Further volumes will introduce Tibetan, Taoist, and Buddhist (Zen) meditation methods.

As you can see, this is a very ambitious undertaking, and I can foresee a number of difficulties both in finance and writing. It will be a new challenge for YMAA and myself, and it will take many years of effort to complete. However, with your support and encouragement, we will complete it, even if it takes longer than anticipated.

This manual will start by briefly introducing in the first two chapters the history of Chi Kung and the fundamental theory. The third and fourth chapters in this volume will introduce the sitting and the standing sets of the Eight Pieces of Brocade.

The Eight Pieces of Brocade is only one of the many Chi Kung health exercises which will be introduced in the later volume: "Chi Kung and Health."

CONTENTS

CHAPTER 1
GENERAL INTRODUCTION

1-1. Introduction

If you study the history of the human race, you will see that a large part of the time has been taken up with war, conquest, killing, and the struggle for power. We have tended to worship as heroes those who could conquer and rule other countries, and we have wrongly educated each new generation to glorify killing and slavery, and to worship power. There have been only relatively short periods when mankind has not been at war, when people could live their lives in peace and tranquility, but it was during these times that people created art, wrote poems, and sought ways to live longer and happier lives.

In their seven thousand years of history, the Chinese people have experienced all possible human suffering and pain. Chinese culture is like a seven thousand year old man who has seen and experienced all of the painful side of human life. Yet through his experience, he has also accumulated a great store of knowledge. China's long spiritual experience cannot be compared to the popular culture of the West, which is the result of centuries of emphasis on the material sciences, money, war, and conquest. If you research Chinese culture through its literature and painting, you will discover that it ranks among the greatest achievements of the human spirit. It reflects mankind's joy and grief, pleasure and sufferings, peace and strife, vitality, sickness, and death.

Coming from this complex cultural and historical background, the Chinese people have long sought ways of living healthy and happy lives. However, while on the one hand the Chinese study themselves spiritually, they also tend to say that everything that happens is destiny, and is pre-arranged by heaven. While holding the fatalistic belief that everything is predetermined, the Chinese also looked for ways to resist the apparent inevitability of sickness and death.

It was with this seemingly contradictory and no-win point of view that the Chinese focused their attention on self-study and self-cultivation. This inward-feeling and looking, this spiritual searching, has become one of the major roots of Chinese culture and medical science. Once Chi, or the internal energy within the human body, was discovered, it was studied very carefully. When the link between the Chi in the human body and the Chi in nature was discovered, the hope soon grew that this Chi was the means whereby man could escape from the trap of sickness and death. When viewed from this historical background, it is not hard to understand why the major part of Chinese culture, other than warfare, was based on the religions of Taoism and Buddhism, and spiritual science.

So many people today are devoting all their efforts to striving for, and even achieving, material wealth, and yet they are suffering spiritually. They wander through their lives, listlessly or frantically, wondering what it is they are missing. Their lives have no meaning or purpose. Many seek temporary release from their pain through drugs. I deeply believe that if these people were to study the spiritual practices which have been developed over these several thousand years, they would find the mental balance which is especially necessary for today's society.

In this chapter we will first define Chi and Chi Kung, and then survey the history of Chi Kung. This will be followed by the story of the creator of the Eight Pieces of Brocade. Finally, Chi Kung theory and training principles will be discussed.

1-2. Definition of Chi and Chi Kung
What is Chi?

In order to understand Chi Kung, you must first understand what Chi is. Chi is the energy or natural force which fills the universe. There are three general types of Chi. Heaven (the sky or universe) has Heaven Chi (Tian Chi), which is made up of the forces which the heavenly bodies exert on the earth, such as sunshine, moonlight, and the moon's affect on the tides. The Earth has Earth Chi (Di Chi), which absorbs the Heaven Chi, and is influenced by it. Man has Human Chi (Zen Chi), which is influenced by the other two. In ancient times, the Chinese believed that it was Heaven Chi which controlled the weather, climate, and natural disasters. When this Chi or energy field loses its balance, it strives to rebalance itself. Then the wind must blow, rain must fall, even tornados and hurricanes must happen in order for the Heaven Chi to reach a new energy balance. Heaven Chi also affects Human Chi, and divination and astrology are attempts to explain this.

Under Heaven Chi, the most important of the three, is the Earth Chi. It is influenced and controlled by the Heaven Chi. For example, too much rain will force a river to flood or change its path. Without rain, the plants will die. The Chinese believe that Earth Chi is made up of lines and patterns of energy, as well as the earth's magnetic field and the heat concealed underground. These energies must also balance, otherwise disasters such as earthquakes will occur. When the Chi of the earth is balanced, plants will grow and animals will prosper. Also, each individual person, animal, and plant has its own Chi field, which always seeks to be balanced. When any individual thing loses its balance, it will sicken, die, and decompose.

You must understand that all natural things, including man, grow within, and are influenced by, the natural cycles of Heaven Chi and Earth Chi. Since you are part of this nature (Tao), you must understand Heaven Chi and Earth Chi. Then you will be able to adjust yourself, when necessary, to fit more smoothly into the natural cycle, and you will learn how to protect yourself from the negative influences in nature. This is the major target of Chi Kung practice.

From this you can see that in order to have a long and healthy life, the first rule is that you must live in harmony with the cycles of nature, and avoid and prevent the negative influences. The Chinese have researched nature for thousands of years. Some of the information on the patterns and cycles of nature has been recorded in books, one of which is the I Ching (Classic of Changes). This book gives the average person formulas to trace when the season will change, when it will snow, when a farmer should plow or harvest. You must remember that nature is always repeating itself. If you observe carefully, you will be able to see many of these routine patterns and cycles caused by the rebalancing of the Chi fields.

Over thousands of years the Chinese have researched the interrelationships of all things in nature, especially in regard to human beings. From this experience, they have created various Chi Kung exercises to help bring the body's Chi circulation into harmony with nature's cycles. This helps to avoid illnesses caused by weather or seasonal changes.

After the long period of research and study, the Chinese also discovered that through Chi Kung practice they were able to strengthen their Chi or internal energy circulation, and slow down the degeneration of the body, gaining not only health but also a longer life. The realization that such things were possible greatly spurred new research.

What is Chi Kung?

From the above discussion you can see that Chi is energy, and is found in heaven, in the earth, and in every living thing. All of these different types of energy interact with each other, and can convert to each other. In China, the word "Kung" is often used instead of "Kung Fu", which means energy and time. Any study or training which requires a lot of energy and time to learn or to accomplish is called Kung Fu. The term can be applied to any special skill or study as long as it requires time, energy, and patience. Therefore, the correct definition of Chi Kung is any training or study dealing with Chi which takes a long time and a lot of effort.

Chi exists in everything, from the largest to the smallest. Since the range of Chi is so vast, the Chinese have divided it into three categories, parallel to the Three Powers (Shan Chai) of Heaven, Earth, and Man. Generally speaking, Heaven Chi is the biggest and the most powerful. This Heaven Chi contains within it the Earth Chi, and within this Heaven and Earth Chi lives man, with his own Chi (Figure 1-1). You can see from the diagram that Human Chi is part of Heaven and Earth Chi. However, since the human beings who research Chi are mainly interested in Human Chi, the term Chi Kung is usually used to refer only to Chi training for people.

As you can see, Chi Kung research should include Heaven Chi, Earth Chi, and Human Chi. Understanding Heaven Chi is very difficult, however, and it was especially so in ancient times when the science was just developing. The major rules and principles relating to Heaven Chi can be found in such books as The Five Elements and Ten Stems, Celestial Stems, and the I Ching.

Many people have become proficient in the study of Earth Chi. They are called Di Li Shy (Geomancy Teachers) or Feng Shui Shy (Wind Water Teachers). These experts use the accumulated body of geomantic knowledge and the I Ching to help people make important decisions such as where and how to build a house, or even where to locate a grave. This profession is still quite common in China.

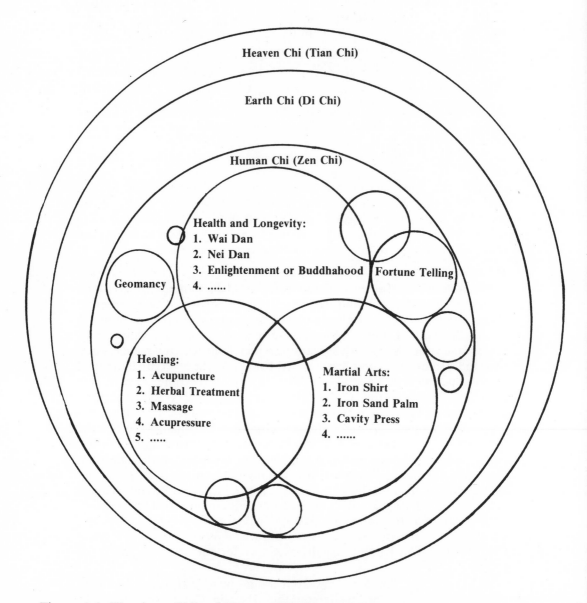

Figure 1-1. The three Chi's of Heaven, Earth, and Man

The Chinese people believe that Human Chi is affected and controlled by Heaven Chi and Earth Chi, and that they in fact determine your destiny. Some people specialize in explaining these connections; they are called Suann Ming Shy (Calculate Life Teachers), or fortune tellers.

Most Chi Kung research has focused on Human Chi. Since Chi is the source of life, if you understand how Chi functions and know how to affect it correctly, you should be able to live a long and healthy life. Many different aspects of Human Chi have been researced, including acupuncture, acupressure, herbal treatment, meditation, and Chi Kung exercises. The use of acupuncture, acupressure, and herbal treatment to adjust Human Chi flow has become the root of Chinese medical science. Meditation and moving Chi Kung exercises are widely used by the Chinese people to improve their health or even to cure certain illnesses. Meditation and Chi Kung exercises serve an additional role in that Taoists and Buddhists use them in their spiritual pursuit of enlightenment and Buddhahood.

You can see that the study of any of the aspects of Chi should be called Chi Kung. However, since the term is usually used today only in reference to the cultivation of Human Chi, we will use it only in this narrower sense to avoid confusion.

1-3. The History of Chi Kung

Chinese Chi Kung history can be divided roughly into three periods. The history of the first period is vague, although it is considered to have started when the I Ching (Book of Changes) was introduced to the Chinese people sometime before 2400 B.C., and to extend until the Han dynasty (206 B.C.) when Buddhism and its meditation methods were imported from India. This led Chi Kung practice and meditation into the second period, the religious Chi Kung era. This period lasted until the Liang dynasty (502-557 A.D.), when it was discovered that Chi Kung could be used for martial purposes, which started the third period of martial Chi Kung. In this third period, different martial Chi Kung styles were created based on theories and principles from Buddhist and Taoist Chi Kung. This period lasted until the overthrow of the Ching dynasty in 1911, when a new era started in which Chinese Chi Kung training is being mixed with Chi Kung practices from India, Japan, and many other countries.

Before the Han Dynasty (before 206 B. C.)

When the I Ching (Book of Changes; 2400 B.C.) was introduced to the Chinese people, they believed that natural energy or power include Tian (Heaven), Di (Earth) and Zen (Man). These were called San Chai (The Three Natural Powers). These three facets of nature have their definite rules and cycles. The rules never change, and the cycles repeat periodically. Therefore, if you could understand the rules and the cycles of Tian Shyr (Heavenly Timing), you would be able to understand natural changes such as the seasons, climate, weather, rain, snow, drought, and all other natural occurrences. Among the natural cycles are those of the day, the month, and the year, as well as cycles of twelve years and sixty years.

If you understand the rules and the structure of the earth, you will be able to understand geography, how plants grow, how rivers move, where the best place to live is, where to build a house and which direction it should face so that it is a healthy place to live, and many other things related to the earth. In China today there are people who make their living in the profession called Di Li (Geomancy) or Feng Shui (Wind Water). Feng Shui is commonly used because the location and character of the wind and water in a landscape are the most important factors in evaluating a location. These professionals help people choose where to live, where to bury their dead, and even how to rearrange or redecorate homes and offices so that they are better places to live and work in.

When you understand Zen Shih (Humans Relations), you will be able to understand the relationship between nature and people, the relationships between people, and the destiny of an individual. If you understand the Three Natural Powers, you will be able to predict natural disasters, the fate of a country, or the future of a person. The Chinese believe that in this universe, it is the Chi, or natural energy, which demonstrates these natural rules and cycles. This natural force decides everything, makes the plants grow, effects the birth of a child, and influences the destiny of a country, or even a person's desires and temperament. This field has generated a profession called Suann Ming (Calculate Life), which is devoted to fortune telling.

It is easy to understand that you were formed and grew under the influence of natural rules and cycles. You are part of nature, and you are channeled into the cycles of nature. If you go against this natural cycle, you will become sick and soon die. If you know the natural cycles and learn how to live with them, you will gain a long and healthy life. That is the meaning of "Tao", which can be translated as "The Natural Way."

Based on the understanding of these principles, the Chinese people figured out a way to calculate the changes of natural Chi. This calculation is called Ba Kua (The Eight Trigrams). From the Eight Trigrams are derived the 64 hexagrams. Therefore, the I Ching was probably the first book which taught the Chinese people about Chi and its variations in nature and man. The relationship of the Three Natural Powers and their Chi variations were later discussed extensively in the book "Chi Far Lun" (Theory of Chi's Variation).

Around 1766-1154 B.C. (the Shang dynasty) Chinese doctors started using stone probes called "Bian Shih" (Figure 1-2) to adjust people's Chi circulation. This is considered the beginning of acupuncture. During the Jou dynasty (1122-934 B.C.), Lao Tzu (Li Erh) described certain breathing techniques in his classic "Tao Te Ching" (Classic on the Virtue of the Tao). Later, "Shih Gi" (Historical Record) in the Spring and Autumn and Warring States Periods (770-221 B.C.) also described more complete methods of breath training. About 300 B.C. the Taoist philosopher Chuang Tzu described the relationship between health and the breath.

During the Chin and Han dynasties (221 B.C. to 220 A.D.), several books were written which discussed the circulation of Chi, such as the Nan Ching (Classic on Disorders) by Bian Chiueh, Gin Guey Yao Liueh (Prescriptions from the Golden Chamber) by Chang Chung-Gieh, and Jou I Chan Ton Chi (A Comparative Study of the Jou (Dynasty) Book of Changes) by Wei Bo-Yang. It can be seen from this list that up to this time, almost all of the publications were written by scholars such as Lao Tzu and Chuang Tzu, or medical doctors such as Bian Chiueh and Wei Bo-Yang.

Characteristics of Chi Kung in this period were:

1. There were two major types of Chi Kung training. One type was used by the Confucian and Taoist scholars, who used it primarily to maintain their health. The other type of Chi Kung was for medical purposes, using needles or exercises to adjust the Chi or to cure illness.

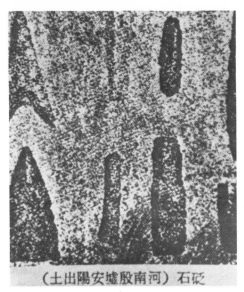

（土出陽安墟殷南河）石砭

Figure 1-2. Acupuncture stone probes (Bian Shih)

2. Except for Taoism, there was almost no religious color to the training.
3. All of the training was passive rather than active, gently improving and maintaining health.

After the Han Dynasty and before the Liang Dynasty (to 502 A. D.)

In China, the Han dynasty was a glorious and peaceful period. It was during the Eastern Han dynasty (c. 58 A.D.) that Buddhism was imported to China from India. Because the Han emperor was a sincere Buddhist, Buddhism soon spread, and became very popular. Many Buddhist meditation and Chi Kung practices, which had been practiced in India for thousands of years, were absorbed into the Chinese culture. The Buddhist temples taught many Chi Kung practices, especially still meditation or Chan (Zen), which marked a new era of Chi Kung practice. Much of the deeper Chi Kung theory and practices which had been developed in India were brought to China. Unfortunately, since the training was directed at attaining Buddhahood, the training practices and theory were recorded in the Buddhist bibles and kept secret. For hundreds of years the religious Chi Kung training was never taught to laymen. Only in this century has it been available to the general populace.

Not long after Buddhism was imported into China, a Taoist by the name of Chang Tao-Ling combined the traditional Taoist principles with Buddhism and created a religion called Tao Jiaw. Many of the meditation methods were a combination of the principles and training methods of both sources.

Since Tibet had its own branch of Buddhism with its own training system and methods of attaining Buddhahood, Tibetan Buddhists were also invited to China to preach. In time, their practices were also absorbed.

In addition to the Chi Kung meditations which were passed down secretly within the monasteries, traditional scholars and physicians continued their Chi Kung research. During the Gin dynasty in the 3rd century A.D., a famous physician named Hua Tor used acupuncture for anesthesia in surgery. The Taoist Juan Gin used the movements of animals to create the Wu Chin Si (Five Animal Sports), which taught people how to increase their Chi circulation. Also, in this period, a physician named Gar Hung mentioned using the mind to lead and increase Chi in his book Bao Poh Tzu . In the period of 420 to 581 A.D. Tao Hung-Gin compiled the Yang Shenn Yen Ming Lu (Records of Nourishing the Body and Extending Life), which showed many Chi Kung techniques.

Characteristics of Chi Kung during this period were:

1. There were three schools of religious Chi Kung which influenced and dominated the Chi Kung practice in this period. These are Indian Buddhism, Tibetan Buddhism, and Taoism.
2. Almost all of the religious Chi Kung practices were kept secret within the monasteries.
3. Religious Chi Kung training worked to escape from the cycle of reincarnation.
4. Relatively speaking, religious Chi Kung theory is harder to understand than the theory of the non-religious Chi Kung, and the training is harder.
5. Chi circulation theory was better understood by this time, so the Chi Kung sets created in this period seem to be more efficient than the older sets.

From the Liang Dynasty to the Late Ching Dynasty (to 1911 A. D.)

During the Liang dynasty (502-557 A.D.) the emperor invited an Indian prince named Da Mo, who was also a Buddhist monk, to preach Buddhism in China. When the emperor decided he did not like his Buddhist theory, the monk retreated to the Shaolin temple. When Da Mo arrived at the Shaolin Temple, he saw that the priests were weak and sick. He decided to shut himself away to ponder the problem. He stayed in seclusion for nine years. When he emerged he wrote two classics: Yi Gin Ching (Muscle/Tendon Changing Classic) and Shii Soei Ching (Marrow Washing Classic). The Muscle/Tendon Changing Classic taught the priests how to gain health and change their physical bodies from weak to strong. The Marrow Washing Classic taught the priests how to use the internal energy or Chi to clean the bone marrow and strengthen the blood and immune system as well as how to energize the brain and attain Buddhahood or enlightenment. Because the Marrow Washing Classic was harder to understand and practice, the training methods were passed down secretly to only a very few disciples in each generation.

After the priests practiced the Muscle/Tendon Changing exercises, they found that not only did they improve their health, but they also greatly increased their strength. When this training was integrated into the martial arts forms, it increased the effectiveness of their techniques. In addition to this martial Chi Kung training, the Shaolin priests also created five animal styles of Kung Fu from watching the way the different animals fight. The animals imitated were the tiger, leopard, dragon, snake, and crane.

Outside of the monastery, development of Chi Kung continued during the Sui and Tang dynasties (581-907 A.D.). Chow Yun-Fan compiled the Chu Bin Yun Hou Lun (Thesis on the Origins and Symptoms of Various Diseases), which is a veritable encyclopedia of Chi Kung methods. He listed 260 different ways of increasing the Chi flow. The Chen Gin Fan (Thousand Gold Prescriptions) by Sun Ssu-Mao described the method of leading Chi, and also described the use of the six sounds. The use of the six sounds to regulate Chi in the internal organs had already been used by the Buddhists and Taoists for some time. Sun Ssu-Mao also introduced a massage system called Lao Tzu's 49 Massage Techniques. Wai Tai Mi Yao (The Extra Important Secret) by Wang Tor discussed the use of breathing and herbal therapies for disorders of Chi circulation.

During the Sung, Gin, and Yuan dynasties (960 -1368 A.D.), Yang Shenn Gieh (Life Nourishing Secrets) by Chang An-Tao discussed several Chi Kung practices. Zu Men Shih Shih (The Confucian Point of View) by Chang Tzu-Huo uses Chi Kung to cure external injuries such as cuts and sprains. Lan Shih Mi Chan (Secret Library of the Orchid Room) by Li Gou uses Chi Kung and herbal remedies for internal disorders. Ge Tzi Yu Lun (A Further Thesis of Complete Study) by Chu Dan-Si provided a theoretical explanation for the use of Chi Kung in curing disease.

During the Sung dynasty (960-1279 A.D.), not long after the Shaolin temple started using Chi Kung in their martial training, Chang San-Feng is believed to have created Tai Chi Chuan. Tai Chi follows a different approach in its use of Chi Kung than does Shaolin. While Shaolin emphasizes Wai Dan (External Elixir) Chi Kung exercises, Tai Chi emphasizes Nei Dan (Internal Elixir) Chi Kung training (see the next section for Wai Dan and Nei Dan).

In 1026 A.D. the famous brass man of acupuncture was built by Dr. Wang Wei-Yi. Before this time, although there were many publications which discussed acupuncture theory, principles, and treatment techniques, there were many disagreements among them, and many points which were unclear. When Dr. Wang built his brass man, he also wrote a book called "Torng Ren Yu Hsieh Jen Jeou Twu" (Illustration of the Brass Man Acupuncture and Moxibustion). He explained the relationship of the 12 organs and the 12 Chi channels, clarified many of the points of confusion, and for the first time systematically organized acupuncture theory and principles. In 1034 he used acupuncture to cure the emperor Ren Tsung. With the support of the emperor, acupuncture flourished. His work contributed greatly to the advancement of Chi Kung and Chinese medicine by giving a clear and systematic idea of the circulation of Chi in the human body.

Later, in the Southern Sung dynasty (1127-1279), Marshal Yeuh Fei was credited with creating several internal Chi Kung exercises and martial arts. It is said that the Eight Pieces of Brocade (Ba Duann Gin) was created by Marshal Yeuh Fei to improve his soldiers' health. He was also known as the creator of the internal martial style Hsing Yi. In addition to that, Eagle Style martial artists also claim that Yeuh Fei was the creator of their style.

From then until the end of the Ching dynasty (1911 A.D.), many other Chi Kung styles were founded. The well known ones include Fu Bu Kung (Tiger Step Kung), Shih Er Chuang (Twelve Postures) and Giaou Far Kung (Beggar Kung). Also in this period, many documents related to Chi Kung were published, such as Bao Shenn Mi Yao (The Secret Important Document of Body Protection) by Tso Yun-Bai, which described moving and stationary Chi Kung practice; Yang Shenn Huo Yu (Brief Introduction to Nourishing the Body) by Chen Gi-Zu, about the three treasures: Jieng (essence), Chi (internal energy), and Shen (spirit). Also, Yi Fan Gi Gieh (The Total Introduction to Medical Prescriptions) by Wong Fan-Yen reviewed and summarized the previously published materials, Nei Kung Twu Shwo (Illustrated Explanation of Nei Kung) by Wang Tzu-Yun presented the Twelve Pieces of Brocade, and also explained the idea of combining both moving and stationary Chi Kung.

In the late Ming dynasty (1640 A.D.) a martial Chi Kung style, For Long Kung (Fire Dragon Kung) was created by the Tai Yang martial stylists. Late in the Ching dynasty (1644-1911 A.D.), the well known internal martial Art style named Ba Kua Chang was created by Tung Hai-Chuan. This style is now gaining in popularity throughout the world.

Before 1911 A.D., Chinese society was still very old fashioned and conservative. Even though China had been expanding its contact with the outside world for the last hundred years, the outside world had little influence beyond the coastal regions. With the overthrow of the Ching dynasty and the founding of the Chinese Republic, the nation started changing as never before. Therefore, we would like to draw a line at 1911 and consider the time since then as a new period. Before we discuss the present period, let us first summarize a few points which marked the characteristics of the previous period:

1. Chi Kung was adapted into the martial arts, and martial Chi Kung styles were created.
2. Chi circulation theory and Chinese acupuncture technologies had reached a peak. More documents were published about medical Chi Kung than about regular Chi Kung exercises.
3. Religious Chi Kung practice remained secret.
4. Chi Kung exercises had become more popular in Chinese society.

From the Late Ching Dynasty to the Present
Since 1911 A.D., Chi Kung practice has entered a new era. Because of the ease of communication in the modern world, Western culture is having a great influence on the Orient. Many Chinese have opened their minds and changed their traditional ideas, especially in Taiwan and Hong Kong. The various Chi Kung styles are now being taught openly, and many formerly secret documents have been published. Modern methods of communication have opened up Chi Kung to a much wider audience than ever before, and people now have the chance to study and understand many different styles. In addition to that, people are now able to compare Chinese Chi Kung to similar arts from other countries such as India, Japan, Korea, and the Middle East. I deeply believe that in the near future Chi Kung will be considered the most exciting and challenging field of research. It is an ancient science just waiting to be investigated with the help of the new technologies now being developed at an almost explosive rate. Anything we can do to speed up this research will greatly help humanity to understand and improve itself.

1-4. History of the Eight Pieces of Brocade
The Eight Pieces of Brocade were created by Marshal Yeuh Fei (Figure 1-3) to improve the health of his soldiers. It is said that originally there were twelve pieces of brocade, but after being passed down from generation to generation for more than eight hundred years, they were edited down to eight pieces. Yeuh Fei is not only credited with being the creator of the Eight Pieces of Brocade, but he is also recognized as the founder of two martial styles: Eagle Claw (an external style) and Hsing I (an internal style). Yeuh Fei is considered one of the wisest and bravest heroes in the history of China, and he is highly respected even today. Before you start practicing this set of Chi Kung exercises which has been benefiting the Chinese people for nearly one thousand years, it is good to first study the background of its creator.

The Sung dynasty in China was a sorrowful time for the Chinese. Wars with the northern barbarians (the Gin race), corruption in business and government, and the specter of starvation constantly oppressed the people. But in the midst of all these troubles there arose a man who showed by the purity of his spirit and ideals that goodness, righteousness, and loyalty were qualities that still lived. For countless generations after

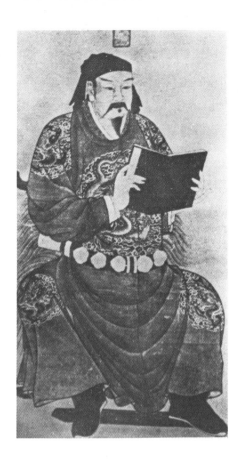

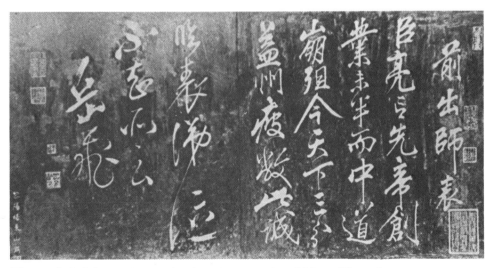

Figure 1-3. Marshal Yeuh Fei and a sample of his calligraphy

his betrayal and murder at the hands of traitors, Marshal Yeuh Fei remains the ideal for the Chinese people of the completely virtuous man. In peace Yeuh Fei was a great scholar of the Chinese classics, in war Yeuh Fei was a brave and shrewd general who skillfully defeated the enemies of his country.

Yeuh Fei was born on February 15th, 1103 A.D. in Tang Yin Hsien, Henan province. While he was being born, a momentous event took place: a large, powerful bird called a perng flew onto the roof and began to make a tremendous noise. The father sensed that the bird's presence was an omen which foretold a tumultuous yet inspired fate or his son; the father thus named his son Fei which in Chinese means "to fly." This reflected the father's belief that his son would fly to great and noble heights as a man.

When Yeuh Fei was but one month old, tragedy struck: the Yellow River flooded. Yeuh Fei's mother saved herself and her infant son by taking refuge in a giant urn; the urn acted as a small boat and took both mother and son to safety. When they reached dry land and the flood had receded, they went back to find that their home and property were totally destroyed.

Yeuh Fei's mother was very poor, but she was a well-educated scholar, and possessed the courage, intelligence, and bravery to raise her son properly while giving him noble ideals. Because they were too poor to pay for an education, Yeuh Fei's mother taught him personally. Each day she taught him how to read and write by drawing figures in the sand. Even though other children had books, paper, and brushes, the poor Yeuh Fei became one of the most educated youngsters in his village; few children could match his scholarship.

In many ways the most important person and the greatest influence on Yeuh Fei's life was his mother. All the ideals that Yeuh Fei lived and died for were taught to him by his mother as they held their own classes using the sand as a blackboard. Without his mother's teachings and example, Yeuh Fei would never have become the brave, intelligent, and loyal leader that he was.

The young Yeuh Fei was a very avid reader. His favorite subjects were history and military theory. The book he admired and studied the most was Suen's Book of Tactics (Suen Tzu Bin Far), a book written by Suen Tzu (c. 220 B.C.) describing the theory and practice of warfare. From this book Yeuh learned important principles which later helped him in his military career.

When Yeuh Fei was a young man he became a tenant farmer for a landlord named Han Chi. After long hours of work he would come home to continue studying with his mother. Yeuh Fei was much admired for this, and for the great physical strength he showed as a young man. As in scholarship, no one could match his natural power and speed.

These admirable qualities were noticed by a certain man in the town called Jou Ton. Jou Ton himself was a scholar an a very good martial artist who had studied in the Shaolin Temple. Seeing that Yeuh Fei possessed many noble qualities, Jou Ton began to teach him martial arts. Martial arts as it was taught to Yeuh Fei was a complete system involving barehand combat, weapons, military tactics, horsemanship, archery, and other related subjects. By constant practice Yeuh Fei mastered everything Jou Ton taught.

When Yeuh Fei was nineteen years old (1122 A.D.) he decided to aid his country by joining the Sung army in its war against the Gin, a nomadic people who had invaded the Northern Sung. The Sung dynasty, which was originally located in northern China, had to move to the south to re-establish itself with a new capital and emperor because the Gin had sacked their old capital and captured their emperor. The Sung dynasty which was invaded is known as the Northern Sung (960-1127 A.D.), while the Sung dynasty that established itself in the South after the Gin invasion is known as the Southern Sung (1127-1279 A.D.). For years the weakened Southern Sung had to pay tribute to the Gin to keep them from attacking further south. When Yeuh Fei joined the army, the Southern Sung was trying to regain its lost land by war.

Yeuh Fei proved himself to be an extraordinary soldier. His wisdom, bravery, and martial skill earned him promotion after promotion so that he became a general after only six years. Later, Yeuh Fei became the commander or marshal of the army that was assigned to fight the Gin. Upon assuming command, he instituted a systematic training program in martial arts for his soldiers. Although some martial training had previously existed, Yeuh Fei was the first to introduce Wushu into the army as a basic requirement before combat. Many times a young man joined the army only to find himself in battle the very next day. After a while, Yeuh's troops, known as Yeuh Jar Chun (Yeuh Family Troop) became a highly efficient and successful fighting unit.

The success of Yeuh's troops can be basically attributed to three things. First, he made all his training strict; the troops were trained in a serious and professional manner. The soldiers were pushed until they excelled in martial arts. Second, Yeuh Fei set up a military organization that was efficient and well run. Third, and most important, Yeuh Fei created for his troops two new styles of Wushu. The first style which he taught to the troops came from his internal training, and led to the creation of Hsing Yi. The second style, which he created out of external Wushu, was Eagle Claw, a style which put a major emphasis on Chin Na. The external style, because it was learned more easily, and because it had immediately practical techniques, made Yeuh's troops successful in battle.

With his highly trained troops Yeuh Fei was in favor of pressing the attack against the Gin. He was so loyal and patriotic that he felt it was shameful for the Sung to pay the Gin tribute. Yeuh Fei constantly felt intense personal agony from the humiliation that his country suffered. With the desire to free his country constantly on his mind, Yeuh Fei on his own initiative advanced his troops against the Gin to win back honor for the Sung.

When Yeuh Fei went into battle, his highly trained troops had many victories as they began to march north. But Yeuh Fei had not yet encountered the Gin commander Wuh Jwu, who himself had never lost a battle. Wuh Jwu's terrifying success was largely due to his main weapon — the feared Kua Tzu Ma. The Kua Tzu Ma was an ancient version of the tank. It was a chariot carrying armored men, drawn by three fully armored horses which were connected by a chain. It was extremely difficult to disable either the horses or the riders, and so they completely dominated the battlefield.

Yeuh Fei had given much thought to defending against the awful Kua Tzu Ma. As in other cases, Yeuh's brilliant military mind came up with a solution. He found that the horses were not protected in one place — their legs; putting armor on the horses' legs would have made them immobile. It was too difficult to attack the horses' legs by conventional arrows and spears, so Yeuh Fei devised two simple but effective weapons: a sword with a hooked end, which was extremely sharp on the inside edge of the hook, and a shield made out of a vine called "rattan" (Tern). This army was called Tern Pai Chun, or "The Rattan Shield Army."

At last, both generals met on a fateful day. When the battle started, Yeuh Fei had the Rattan Shield Army crouching very low in the path of the Kua Tzu Ma. Before the chariots could reach the soldiers, they ran into obstacles such as ditches and upright spears which Yeuh Fei had had set up. Once these slowed down the chariots, Yeuh Fei's soldiers, who were mainly on foot, could move against the enemy with more ease. As the chariots advanced, the crouching men hooked and cut the legs of the horses, making them fall. It was impossible for the horses to trample the crouching men because the shields were greased, and the horses slipped every time they put their feet on them. When the crouching soldiers attacked the horses they only had to cripple one animal to stop a chariot. Once a chariot was stopped, other soldiers surrounded it and killed the riders. On that day Yeuh Fei scored a military victory which lives today in history and legend.

Yeuh Fei then proceeded north, regaining lost territory and defeating such Gin generals as the Tiger King and Great Dragon. But while Yeuh Fei was gaining his country's honor back, the Gin leaders successfully bribed one of the most infamous men in Chinese history — Chin Kua — to stop Yeuh Fei. Chin Kua was at that time the prime minister, and the most influential man at the emperor's corrupt court.

While Yeuh Fei's army moved north, Chin Kua, to achieve his evil act, decided to send an imperial order with the emperor's official golden seal (Gin Pie), asking Yeuh Fei to come back. According to tradition, a general fighting on the front line had the option of refusing an order of retreat. Chin Kua was counting on Yeuh Fei's patriotic sense of loyalty to the emperor to get him back. To ensure Yeuh Fei's return, Chin Kua sent twelve gold-sealed orders in one day; so much pressure made Yeuh Fei return.

When Yeuh Fei returned he was immediately imprisoned. Because Chin Kua feared that any sort of trial would reveal Yeuh Fei's innocence, he ordered an officer named Ho Juh to thoroughly investigate Yeuh Fei's life in an attempt to find some excuse for the imprisonment. Ho Juh searched and searched, but he found nothing. Although a powerful general, Yeuh Fei had never abused his position for bad purposes. Ho Juh found that Yeuh Fei had lived a spartan life, and had fewer possessions than a peasant. When Ho Juh returned to Chin Kua, he reported only one fact of significance. When Yeuh Fei joined the army his mother tatooed on his back a certain phrase: "Be loyal and pure to serve your country" (Ginn Chung Pau Kuo).

With such an honest general as Yeuh Fei, Chin Kua had only one alternative—to have his food poisoned. Thus was the noble general viciously betrayed by his own countrymen. Without the glory and honor that was his right, Yeuh Fei died in jail on January 27, 1142 A.D. (December 9, 1141 A.D. Chinese calendar). Yeuh Fei was thirty-eight years old. Later, Yeuh Fei's adopted son, Yeuh Yun, and Yeuh Fei's top assistant, Chang Shien, were also killed.

For twenty years Yeuh Fei was officially considered a criminal. But in 1166 A.D. a new and better government and emperor (Xiao Zong) took control. They refused to believe in the treachery of Yeuh Fei, and relocated his grave to the beautiful West Lake in Hangzhou. In front of the grave are stone statues of Chin Kua and his wife (Figure 1-4), kneeling in repentance and shame before Yeuh Fei. These statues have to be replaced periodically, because many of the people who come to worship at the grave will deface or damage them out of anger at their treachery.

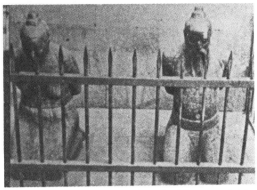

Figure 1-4. Statues of Chin Kua and his wife

Emperor Xiao Zong bestowed upon Yeuh Fei a new name which symbolized what he always was and always will be: Yeuh Wu Mu — "Yeuh, the righteous and respectable warrior."

1-5. Chi Kung Theory and Training Categories

Many people think that Chi Kung is a difficult subject to understand. In some ways, this is true. However, you must understand one thing: regardless of how difficult the Chi Kung theory and practice of a particular style are, the basic theory and principles are very simple and remain the same for all of the Chi Kung styles. The basic theory and principles are the roots of the entire Chi Kung practice. If you understand these roots, you will be able to grasp the key of the practice and grow. All of the Chi Kung styles originated from this root, but each one has blossomed differently.

In this section, we will discuss these basic theories and principles. With this knowledge as a foundation, you will be able to understand not only what you should be doing, but also why you are doing it. Naturally, it is impossible to discuss all of the basic Chi Kung ideas in such a short section. However, it will offer the beginner the key to open the gate into the spacious, four thousand year old garden of Chinese Chi Kung.

Chi and Man:

In order to use Chi Kung to improve and maintain your health, you must know that there is Chi in your body, and you must understand how it circulates, and what you can do to insure that the circulation is smooth and strong.

After reading the above discussion, you know that Chi is energy. It is a requirement for life. The Chi in your body cannot be seen, but it can be felt. This Chi can make your body feel too positive (too Yang) or too negative (too Yin).

Imagine that your physical body is a machine, and your Chi is the current that makes it run. Without the current the machine is dead and unable to function. It is the same with Chi in your body. For example, when you pinch yourself, you feel pain. Have you ever thought "how do I feel pain?" You might answer that it is because you have a nervous system in your body which perceives the pinch and sends a signal to the brain. However, you should understand that there is more to it than that. The nervous system is material, and if it didn't have energy circulating in it, it wouldn't function. Chi is the energy which makes the nervous system and the other parts of your body work. When you pinch your skin, that area is stimulated and the Chi field is disturbed. Your brain is designed to sense this and other disturbances, and to interpret the cause.

The Chi in your body is divided into two categories: Managing Chi (Ying Chi)(which is often called Nutritive Chi) and Guardian Chi (Wei Chi). The Managing Chi is the energy which has been sent to the organs so that they can function. The Guardian Chi is the energy which has been sent to the surface of the body to form a shield to protect you from negative outside influences such as cold. In order to keep yourself healthy, you must learn how to manage these two Chi's efficiently so they can serve you well.

How does Chi circulate in the body? Chinese doctors discovered long ago that the human body has twelve major channels and eight vessels through which the Chi circulates. The twelve channels are like rivers which distribute Chi throughout the body, and also connect the extremities (fingers and toes) to the internal organs. We would like to point out here that the "internal organs" of Chinese medical theory do not necessarily correspond to the physical organs as understood in the West, but rather to a set of clinical functions similar to each other, and related to the organ system. The eight vessels, which are often referred to as the extraordinary vessels, function like reservoirs and regulate the distribution and circulation of Chi in your body.

When the Chi in the eight reservoirs is full and strong, the Chi in the rivers is strong and will be regulated efficiently. When there is stagnation in any of these twelve channels or rivers, the Chi which flows to the body's extremities and to the internal organs will be abnormal, and illness may develop. You should understand that every channel has its particular Chi flow strength, and every channel is different. All of these different levels of Chi strength are affected by your mind, the weather, the time of day, the food you have eaten, and even your mood. For example, when the weather is dry the Chi in the lungs will tend to be more positive than when it is moist. When you are angry, the Chi flow in your liver channel will be abnormal. The Chi strength in the different channels varies throughout the day in a regular cycle, and at any particular time one channel is strongest. For example, between 11 AM and 1 PM the Chi flow in the heart channel is the strongest. Furthermore, the Chi level of the same organ can be different from one person to another.

Whenever the Chi flow in the twelve rivers or channels is not normal, the eight reservoirs will regulate the Chi flow and bring it back to normal. For example, when you experience a sudden shock, the Chi flow in the bladder immediately becomes deficient. Now, normally the reservoir will immediately regulate the Chi in this channel so that you recover from the shock. However, if the reservoir Chi is also deficient, or if the effect of the shock is too great and there is not enough time to regulate the Chi, the bladder will suddenly contract, causing unavoidable urination.

When a person is sick because of an injury, his Chi level tends to be either too positive (excessive, Yang) or too negative (deficient, Yin). A Chinese physician would either use a prescription of herbs to adjust the Chi, or else he would insert acupuncture needles at various spots on the channels to inhibit the flow in some channels and stimulate the flow in others, so that balance can be restored. However, there is another alternative, and that is to use certain physical and mental exercises to adjust the Chi. In other words, to use Chi Kung.

Chi Kung Categories:
As you can see, it is very important to keep the Chi or internal energy

circulating smoothly in your body. Many different kinds of Chi Kung exercises have been created to achieve this, but they can generally be categorized into four groups according to the main purpose of the training:

1. Maintaining Health

The main purpose of the Chi Kung styles in this category is to first gain mental and spiritual calmness, peace, and balance. With this mental balance, you can then engage in moving exercises which maintain the smoothness and balance of the Chi circulation. This category uses both still meditation and moving meditative exercises.

It is believed that many illnesses are caused by mental and emotional excesses. These emotions use up Chi, and cause stagnation in the channels and organ systems, which causes you to get sick. For example, depression can cause stomach ulcers and indigestion. Anger will cause the liver to malfunction. Sadness will cause compression and tightness in the lungs, and fear can disturb the normal functioning of the kidneys and bladder. Chinese Chi Kung practitioners therefore realized that if you want to avoid illness, the first step is to balance and relax your thoughts. This is called "regulating the mind." When your mind is calm, and you are emotionally neutral, your Chi will automatically regulate itself and correct imbalances.

In the still meditation used for maintaining health, the major part of the training is getting rid of thoughts so that the mind is clear and calm. When you become peaceful and calm, the flow of thoughts and emotions slows down, and you feel mentally and emotionally neutral. This kind of meditation can be thought of as practicing emotional self-control. When you are in this "no thought" state, you become very relaxed, and can even relax deep down into your internal organs. When your body is this relaxed, your Chi will naturally flow smoothly and strongly, clearing obstructions in the channels and maintaining your health. This kind of still meditation was very common in ancient Chinese scholarly society.

Chinese physicians discovered that certain movements or exercises increased the Chi circulation around the internal organs. Some of these movements are similar to movements which are characteristic of certain animals. It is clear that in order for an animal to survive in the wild, it must have an instinct for how to protect its body. Part of this instinct is concerned with how to build up its Chi, and how to keep its Chi from being lost. We humans have lost many of these instincts over the years that we have been separating ourselves from natur. One typical set of these Chi Kung exercises which is still practiced today is called "Wu Chin Si" (Five Animal Sports). Another is the Eight Pieces of Brocade.

Over the thousands of years of observing nature and themselves, some Chi Kung practitioners went even deeper. They realized that your body's Chi circulation changes with the seasons, and that it is a good idea to help the body out in these periodic adjustments. They also noticed that during each season, different organs had characteristic problems. For example, in the beginning of Fall the lungs have to adapt to the colder and dryer air that you are breathing. While this adjusting is going on, the lungs are susceptible to disturbance, so your lungs may feel uncomfortable and you may catch colds easily.

Your digestive system is also affected during seasonal changes. Your appetite may increase, or you may have diarrhea. When the temperature goes down, your kidneys and bladder will start to give you trouble. For example, because the kidneys are stressed, you may feel pain in the back.

Focusing on these seasonal Chi disorders, the meditators created a set of movements which can be used to speed up the body's adjustment. These Chi Kung exercises will be introduced in a later volume.

2. Curing Sickness

Chinese doctors discovered through experience that some of the movements could not only maintain health, but could also cure certain illnesses. Using their medical knowledge of Chi circulation, they researched until they had found many movements which could help cure various illnesses and health problems. Naturally, many of the them were not unlike the ones used to maintain health. This is not surprising, since many illnesses are caused by unbalanced Chi. When this stagnation continues for a long period of time, the organs will start to be affected, and may be physically damaged. As a matter of fact, as long as your sickness is limited to the level of Chi stagnation and there is no physical organ damage, the Chi Kung exercises used for maintaining health can be used to readjust your Chi circulation and treat the problem.

However, if the sickness is already so serious that the physical organs start to fail, then the situation has become critical. In this case, a specific treatment is necessary. The treatment can be acupuncture, herbs, or even an operation. Some Chi Kung exercises are designed to speed up the healing, or sometimes even to cure the sickness. For example, ulcers and asthma can be cured with some simple exercises. Recently in both mainland China and Taiwan, certain Chi Kung exercises have been shown to be effective in treating certain kinds of cancer.*

Acupressure or Chi Kung Massage is also commonly used instead of needles to adjust the Chi imbalance. This is done mostly by Chi Kung experts who are able to use their body's Chi to adjust the patient's Chi through touch or acupressure. This is seen in Chinese Chi Kung healing practices and Japanese Shiatsu massage.

3. Prolonging Life

The two preceding categories either maintain the health that a person already has, or else treat illnesses once they appear. The theories and the principles for these categories are simple, and the training is conservative. Many Chinese Chi Kung practitioners were not satisfied with this, and searched for a way that would not only maintain health, but would also increase the Chi circulation and strengthen the organs. In this more aggressive approach to Chi Kung they attempted to find a way to overcome the normal course of nature. They refused to accept that the length of a person's life is set according to destiny. They believed that if they understood the course of nature (Tao) completely, they would be able to find a way to lengthen their lives. This category of Chi Kung training is practiced mostly by Buddhists and Taoists.

Over the more than nineteen hundred years of research, the religious meditators have discovered the way to slow down the degeneration of the organs, which is the key to obtaining a long life. There have been many

---

* There are many reports in popular and professional literature of using Chi Kung to help or even cure many illnesses, including cancer. Many cases have been discussed in the Chinese Chi Kung journals. One book which describes the use of Chi Kung to cure cancer is "New Chi Kung for Preventing and Curing Cancer" (新氣功防治癌症)by Yeh Ming, Chinese Yoga Publications, Taiwan, 1986.

Buddhists and Taoist who have lived more than 150 years. In Taoist society it is said: "One hundred and twenty means dying young."(1)

Unfortunately, all of this Chi Kung training has been passed down secretly in the monasteries. It was not until the last twenty years that these secret theories and training methods were revealed to the outside world. An important part of this training to prolong life is Marrow Washing Chi Kung. The basic idea of Marrow Washing Chi Kung is to keep the Chi circulating in your marrow so that the marrow stays clean and healthy.

Your bone marrow manufactures most of your blood cells. The blood cells bring nourishment to the organs and all the other cells of the body, and also take waste products away. When your blood is healthy and functions properly, your whole body is well-nourished and healthy, and can resist disease effectively. When the marrow is clean and fresh, it manufactures an enormous number of healthy blood cells which will do their job properly. Your whole body will stay healthy, and the organs will not degenerate.

Although the theory is simple, the training is very difficult. You must first learn how to build up your Chi and fill up your eight Chi vessels, and then you must know how to lead this Chi into the bone marrow to "wash" the marrow. However, except for Taoist and Buddhist monks, there are very few people who have lived more than 150 years. The reason for this is that the training process is long and hard. You must have a pure mind and a simple lifestyle so that you can concentrate entirely on the training. Without a peaceful life, your training will not be effective. This is why the Taoist and Buddhist monks hide themselves in the mountains. Unfortunately, this is simply not possible for the average person.

4. Martial Arts

In the Liang dynasty, martial artists started to use Chi Kung to increase the effectiveness of their offense and defense. Such training can also help to improve health. However, some martial artists will even use certain Chi Kung practices which they know will harm their health, if these practices will improve some aspect of their fighting ability. An example of this kind of training is Iron Sand Palm.

5. Enlightenment or Buddhahood

The Taoists and Buddhists use Chi Kung to reach a level of attainment far beyond the average person's. They are striving for enlightenment, or what the Buddhists refer to as Buddhahood. They are looking for a way to lift themselves above the normal human suffering, and to escape from the cycle of continual reincarnation. In order to reach this stage, Marrow Washing Chi Kung training is necessary. This enables them to lead Chi to the forehead, where the spirit resides, and raise the brain to a higher energy state. This will be discussed further in the Marrow Washing Chi Kung book.

1-6. Chi Kung Training

Generally speaking, all Chi Kung practices, according to theory and training, can be divided into two general categories: Wai Dan (External

---

(1). "一百二十謂之夭"

Elixir) and Nei Dan (Internal Elixir). In this section, we will discuss the theories of these two categories. Once you understand these theories, you have built the root of most of the Chinese Chi Kung practices.

Wai Dan (External Elixir)

As previously mentioned, the human body has twelve major Chi channels (Gin), which can be compared to rivers. Six of these are connected to the fingers, and the other six are connected to the toes. All of these twelve are connected to the internal organs. The body also has eight Chi vessels which serve as reservoirs, and regulate the Chi in the channels. Millions of tiny channels (Lou) carry Chi from the major channels to every part of the body, from the skin to the bone marrow. Whenever the Chi is stagnant in any of the twelve major channels, the related organ will receive an incorrect amount of Chi. This will cause the organ to malfunction, or at least to degenerate sooner than normal, and this in turn will cause illness and premature aging. Just as a machine needs the correct amount of current to run properly, your organs must have the right amount of Chi to function well. Therefore, the most basic way to maintain the health of the organs is to keep the Chi flow strong and smooth. This is the idea upon which Wai Dan (External Elixir) Chi Kung is based.

The theory is very simple. When you do the Wai Dan exercises you concentrate your attention on your limbs. As you exercise, the Chi builds up in your arms and legs. When the Chi potential in your limbs builds to a high enough level, the Chi will flow through the channels, clearing any obstructions and nourishing the organs. This is the main reason that a person who works out or has a physical job is generally healthier than someone who sits around all day.

There are many available Wai Dan Chi Kung sets. A typical one is Da Mo's Muscle/Tendon Changing Classic (Yi Gin Ching). In this set, the practitioner slightly tenses up the local limb muscles, such as in the wrist, and then relaxes completely. Through this repeating tensing and relaxing, the Chi is built up to a higher concentration. When the practitioner finishes the exercise and relaxes, the accumulated Chi flows back to the organs.

There are other Wai Dan sets which, in addition to tensing and relaxing the muscles, also move the arms and legs into specific positions so that the muscles around certain organs are also stretched and then relaxed. This increases the Chi circulation around and in the organs more directly than the Muscle/Tendon Changing Classic does. For example, you may repeatedly raise your arms over your head and then lower them. This extends and stretches the muscles around the lungs. This extension and releasing gently massages the lungs and stimulates the Chi and blood flow there. A typical set of Wai Dan which uses both stationary and moving exercises is the Eight Pieces of Brocade.

Many Chi Kung beginners mistakenly believe that since Wai Dan Chi Kung theory and training are simple, these sets are only for beginners. However, most people who train Nei Dan Chi Kung later come back to Wai Dan, and combine the two to increase their control over their Chi. An example of this is Tai Chi Chi Kung. While the sitting meditation is purely Nei Dan, the movements of the Tai Chi solo sequence and the Chi Kung sets are a combination of both Nei Dan and Wai Dan.

Nei Dan (Internal Elixir)

In the higher levels of Chi Kung practice, the theory and principles are more difficult to understand. It is not just that the training is harder. Another problem is that the Nei Dan Chi Kung practices have been passed down more secretly than the Wai Dan. When Nei Dan practice reached to the highest level such as Marrow Washing Chi Kung, it was passed down only to a few disciples. There are a number of reasons for this:

1. Nei Dan is hard to understand, so only the disciples who were intelligent and wise enough to understand it were taught.
2. Nei Dan practice can be dangerous. Inaccurate practice may cause crippling, paralysis, or even death. This can happen especially to the disciple who does not understand the what, why, and how of his practice.
3. In most of the Nei Dan Chi Kung training a disciple must learn and experience directly from a master. Chi Kung is learned and practiced from feeling and sensation. This feeling must be obtained from a master. If the practitioner tries to figure it out by himself, he may possibly get lost. In some cases, he may even cause his own death.
4. In order to reach the higher levels of Nei Dan Chi Kung, you must conserve your Jieng (Essence) and restrain your sex life. You must also spend a lot of time in practice, which makes normal married life impossible. Not only that, in order to reach spiritual balance, you must train yourself to be emotionally neutral and independent. In ancient times, in order to preserve your Jieng (Essence) and have a peaceful environment for your training, you almost had to go away to the mountains and become a hermit, or else become a monk in a monastery.

Even though Nei Dan is difficult to understand and practice, it is still practiced by many non-priests and Chi Kung practitioners in the everyday environment. However, they can only reach a certain level of achievement.

Generally speaking, Nei Dan is a Chi Kung practice in which the Chi is built up inside the body first, and then spread out to the limbs. Nei Dan can be broken down into several categories according to the purpose and depth of training. Generally, after the Chi is built up internally, a Nei Dan Chi Kung practitioner will circulate the Chi throughout his body. Nei Dan includes three paths of Chi circulation: Fire, Wind, and Water.

The Fire Path

The Fire path in Chi Kung is the most fundamental Nei Dan practice among the three. This path is used both by Chi Kung practitioners and martial artists. In the Fire Path, a practitioner usually builds his Chi in the Dan Tien (Field of Elixir) through either abdominal breathing or purely through thinking. When the Chi is built up to a level, he will use his mind to lead the Chi to circulate through the Conception and Governing Vessels (Ren Mei and Du Mei). This path starts at the Dan Tien, passes down to the Huiyin and the tailbone, follows the spine up the back, passes over the crown of the head, moves down the front of the body back to the Dan Tien to complete the cycle (Figure 1-5). This Fire Path is the way Chi routinely circulates in the average person. When there is excess Chi added to this path, there is excess heat (fire).

The Governing Vessel is a major Chi reservoir which also governs or influences the twelve Chi channels or rivers. When the Chi in the Conception and Governing Vessels is strong, the Chi circulation in the

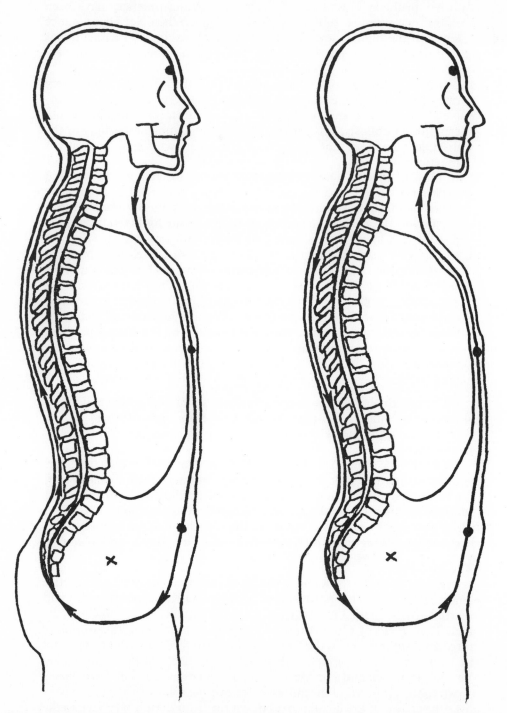

Figure 1-5. The Fire Path of Chi circulation   Figure 1-6. The Wind Path of Chi circulation

twelve organ channels will also be strong and thus benefit the body. However, you must understand one thing: the organ Chi should not be excessive (Yang) or deficient (Yin). When too much Chi is supplied to the organs, it will overheat the organs and speed their degeneration, just as too much sunshine on your skin will cause it to age faster. Therefore, even though this Fire Nei Dan is the simplest of the three practices, if you are not able to sense your organs' Chi level, you might cause problems.

Once a practitioner has opened the circulation path through the Conception and Governing Vessels, he is said to have completed Small Circulation (Shao Jou Tian). He then leads the Chi to the extremities to open the channels in the limbs and also to supply Chi to the skin and the bone marrow. When he is able to do this, he has completed Large Circulation (Da Jou Tian).

The Wind Path

In Wind Path Chi circulation, once the Chi is built up in the Dan Tien, the practitioner will lead the Chi to circulate in the opposite direction as he did with the Fire Path (Figure 1-6). There are many reasons for doing this:

1. To cut down the excess Chi circulation (Fire) to the internal organs.
2. To slow down the natural Chi circulation in the Conception and Governing Vessels if they have become too positive due to sickness, injury, or any other reason.
3. One of the Chi Kung practices is to raise up the Pre-birth Chi (Jieng Chi or Water Chi) generated in the lower Dan Tien to cool down the Post-birth Chi (food and air Chi, or Fire Chi) which is generated in the middle Dan Tien at the solar plexus. The Wind Path is the way to do this.

The Water Path

Water path Chi Kung, which goes through the inside of the spine, is probably one of the highest levels of Chi Kung practice. Once you have built your Pre-birth Chi in the Dan Tien, you use your mind and special training to lead the Chi into the Thrusting Channel (Chong Mei), the Chi reservoir which is located in the marrow of the spine (Figure 1-7). Marrow Washing generates Chi through a different method than the other forms of Chi Kung. Its approach is to convert semen into Chi. This will be discussed in a later volume. The Chi which has been generated by either method is led to the brain to energize the brain and spirit (Shen). The energized mind is then able to adjust the Chi level in the organs and other parts of the body. This Chi Kung practice is difficult to do, but once competence has been achieved it is the most efficient. It is reported that priests who reach this level are able to slow down the aging process to a minimum, and some are able to live over two hundred years.

Marrow Washing Chi Kung has been kept top secret within the Taoist and Buddhist societies. Not only does it enable them to live long and healthy lives, but it is also involved with how they work to reach enlightenment or Buddhahood. Enlightenment or Buddhahood is the final goal of a priest who is looking for the eternal spiritual life.

The Water Path way enables you to reduce the excess fire which most people build up, however the training is the hardest both to practice and to understand.

Conclusion:

Before we finish this section, we would like to conclude the discussion with the following thoughts:

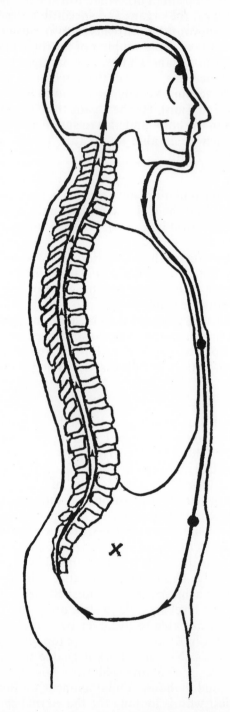

Figure 1-7. The Water Path of Chi circulation

1. Wai Dan Chi Kung is a practice in which Chi is built up in the limbs and then flows to the organs, while in Nei Dan practice the Chi is built up in the body and then spread out to the limbs. Wai Dan practice is mostly physical while Nei Dan practice is primarily mental.
2. Wai Dan is commonly done through muscle tension and relaxation exercises. Wai Dan can also be done with movement of the limbs. Nei Dan can be done either through Dan Tien exercises or simply through thinking.
3. Massage, acupuncture, and acupressure are considered Wai Dan because they rely on outside assistance to adjust the Chi balance.
4. Nei Dan can be dangerous while Wai Dan is usually safe.

Because this book focuses on Wai Dan Chi Kung, this section serves only as a general introduction, and all of the above discussions have necessarily been brief. Interested readers should refer to other documents and books which will be published by YMAA.

1-7. How to Use This Book

When you practice any Chi Kung, you must first ask: What, Why, and How. "What" means: "What am I looking for?" "What do I expect?" and "What should I do?" Then you must ask: "Why do I need it?" "Why does it work?" "Why must I do it this way instead of that way?." Finally, you must determine: "How does it work?" "How much have I advanced toward my goal?" And "How will I be able to advance further?"

It is very important to understand what you are practicing, and not just automatically repeat what you have learned. Understanding is the root of any work. With understanding you will be able to know your goal. Once you know your goal, your mind can be firm and steady. With this understanding, you will be able to see why something has happened, and what the principles and theories behind it are. Without all of this, your work will be done blindly, and it will be a long and painful process. Only when you are sure what your target is and why you need to reach it should you raise the question of how you are going to do it. The answers to all of these questions form the root of your practice, and will help you to avoid the wondering and confusion that uncertainty brings. If you keep this root, you will be able to apply the theory and make it grow — you will know how to create. Without this root, what you learn will be only branches and flowers, and in time they will wither.

In China there is a story about an old man who was able to change a piece of rock into gold. One day, a boy came to see him and asked for his help. The old man said: "Boy! What do you want? Gold? I can give you all of the gold you want." The boy replied: "No, Master, what I want is not your gold, what I want is the trick of how to change the rock into gold!" When you just have gold, you can spend it all and become poor again. If you have the trick of how to make gold, you will never be poor. For the same reason, when you learn Chi Kung you should learn the theory and principle behind it, not just the practice. Understanding theory and principle will not only shorten your time of pondering and practice, but also enable you to practice most efficiently.

One of the hardest parts of the training process is learning how to actually do the forms correctly. Every Chi Kung movement has its special meaning and purpose. In order to make sure your movements or forms are correct, it is best to work with the tape and book together. There are some important things which you may not be able to pick up from reading, but once you see them, they will be clear. An example is the transition movements between the forms. Naturally, there are other important ideas which are impossible to take the time to explain in the videotape, such as the theory and principles; these can only be explained in the book. It cannot be denied that under the tutelage of a master you can learn more quickly and perfectly than is possible using only tapes and books. What you are missing is the master's experience. However, if you ponder carefully and practice patiently and perseveringly, you will be able to fill up this void through your own experience and practice. This book and tape were designed for self-instruction. You will find that they will serve you as a key to enter into the field of Chi Kung.

To conclude, you must practice perseveringly and patiently. You need a strong will and a great deal of patience and self-discipline. You may have already found that there are many different versions of the Eight Pieces of Brocade available on the market. Do not be confused by all of these versions. You should understand that it does not matter which version you practice, the basic theory and principles remain the same. The most important thing of all is to understand the poems and songs which have been passed down through generations. These poems and songs are the root of the training, so please study them carefully.

CHAPTER 2
CHI KUNG TRAINING THEORY

2-1. Introduction

Before you start your Chi Kung training, you must first understand the three treasures of life — Jieng (Essence), Chi (internal energy), and Shen (spirit) — as well as their interrelationship. If you lack this understanding, you are missing the root of Chi Kung training, as well as the basic idea of Chi Kung theory. The main goals of Chi Kung training are to learn how to retain your Jieng, strengthen and smooth your Chi flow, and enlighten your Shen. To reach these goals you must learn how to regulate the body (Tyau Shenn), regulate the mind (Tyau Hsin), regulate the breathing (Tyau Shyi), regulate the Chi (Tyau Chi), and regulate the Shen (Tyau Shen).

Regulating the body includes understanding how to find and build the root of the body as well as of the individual forms you are practicing. To build a firm root, you must know how to keep your center, how to balance your body, and most important of all, how to relax so that the Chi can flow.

Regulating the mind involves learning how to keep your mind calm, peaceful, and centered, so that you can judge situations objectively and lead Chi to the desired places. The mind is the main key to success in Chi Kung practice.

To regulate your breathing, you must learn how to breathe so that your breathing and your mind mutually correspond and cooperate. When you breathe this way, your mind will be able to attain peace more quickly, and therefore concentrate more easily on leading the Chi.

Regulating the Chi is one of the ultimate goals of Chi Kung practice. In order to regulate your Chi effectively, you must first have regulated your body, mind, and breathing. Only then will your mind be clear enough to sense how the Chi is distributed in your body, and understand how to adjust it.

For Buddhist priests, who seek the enlightenment of the Buddha, regulating the Shen is the final goal of Chi Kung. This enables them to maintain a neutral, objective perspective of life, and this perspective is the eternal life of the Buddha. The average Chi Kung practitioner has lower goals. He raises his Shen in order to increase his concentration and enhance his vitality. This makes it possible for him to lead Chi effectively to his entire body so that it carries out the managing and guarding duties. This maintains his health and slows down the aging process.

If you understand these few things you will be able to quickly enter into the field of Chi Kung. Without all of these important elements, your training will be ineffective and your time will be wasted.

2-2. Three Treasures — Jieng, Chi, and Shen

Before you start any Chi Kung training, you must first understand the three treasures (San Bao): Jieng (Essence), Chi (internal energy), and Shen (spirit). They are also called the three origins or the three roots (San Yuan), because they are considered the origins and roots of your life. Jieng means the Essence, the most original and refined part of every thing. Jieng exists in everything. It represents the most basic part of anything which shows its characteristics. Sperm is called Jieng Tzu, which means "Essence of the Son", because it contains the Jieng of the father which is passed on to his son (or daughter) and becomes the son's Jieng. Jieng is the original source of every living thing, and it determines the nature and characteristics of that thing. It is the root of life.

Chi is the internal energy of your body. It is like the electricity which passes through a machine to keep it running. Chi comes either from the conversion of the Jieng which you have received from your parents, or from the food you eat and the air you breathe.

Shen is the center of your mind, the spirit of your being. It is what makes you human, because animals do not have a Shen. The Shen in your body must be nourished by your Chi or energy. When your Chi is full, your Shen will be enlivened.

These three elements are interrelated in a number of ways. Chinese meditators and Chi Kung practitioners believe that the body contains two general types of Chi. The first type is called Pre-birth Chi, and it comes from converted Original Jieng, which you get from your parents at conception. The second type, which is called Post-birth Chi, is drawn from the Jieng of the food and air we take in. When this Chi flows or is led to the brain, it can energize the Shen and soul. This energized and raised Shen is able to lead the Chi to the entire body.

Each one of these three elements or treasures has its own root. You must know the roots so that you can strengthen and protect your three treasures.

1. There are many kinds of Jiengs which your body requires. Except for the Jieng which you inherent from your parents, which is called Original Jieng (Yuan Jieng), all other Jiengs must be obtained from food, air, or even the energy surrounding you. Among all of these Jiengs, Original Jieng is the most important one. It is the root and the seed of your life, and your basic strength. If your parents were strong and healthy, your Original Jieng will be strong and healthy, and you will have a strong foundation on which to grow. The Chinese people believe that in order to stay healthy and live a long life, you must protect and maintain this Jieng. It is like money which you have invested in a bank. You can live off the interest for a long time, but if you withdraw the principal and spend it, you will have nothing left.

   The root of Original Jieng (Yuan Jieng) before your birth was in your parents. After birth this Original Jieng stays in its residence — the kidneys, which are considered the root of your Jieng. When you keep this root strong, you will have sufficient Original Jieng to supply to your body. Although you cannot increase the amount of Jieng you have, Chi Kung training can improve the quality of your Jieng. Chi Kung can also teach you how to convert your Jieng into Original Chi more efficiently, and how to use this Chi effectively.

2. Chi is converted both from the Jieng which you have inherited from your parents and from the Jieng which you draw from the food and air you take in. Chi which is converted from the Original Jieng which you have inherited is called Original Chi.* Just as Original Jieng is the most important type of Jieng, Original Chi is the most important type of Chi. It is pure and of high quality, while the Chi from food and air may make your body too positive or too negative, depending on how and where you absorb it. When you retain and protect your Original Jieng, you will be able to generate Original Chi in a pure, continuous stream. As a Chi Kung practitioner, you must know how to convert your Original Jieng into Original Chi in a smooth, steady stream.

Since your Original Chi comes from your Original Jieng, they both have the kidneys for their root.

When your kidneys are strong, the Original Jieng is strong, and the Original Chi converted from this Original Jieng will also be full and strong. This Chi resides in the lower Dan Tien in your abdomen. Once you learn how to convert your Original Jieng, you will be able to supply your body with all the Chi it needs.

3. Shen is the force which keeps you alive. It has no substance, but it gives expression and appearance to your Jieng. Shen is also the control tower for the Chi. When your Shen is strong, your Chi is strong and you can lead it efficiently. The root of Shen (spirit) is your mind (Yi, or intention). When your brain is energized and stimulated, your mind will be more aware and you will be able to concentrate more intensely. Also, your Shen will be raised. Advanced Chi Kung practitioners believe that your brain must always be sufficiently nourished by your Chi. It is the Chi which keeps your mind clear and concentrated. With an abundant Chi supply, the mind can be energized, and can raise the Shen and enhance your vitality.

The deeper levels of Chi Kung training include the conversion of Jieng into Chi, which is then led to the brain to raise the Shen. This process is called "Huan Jieng Bu Nao" and means "return the Jieng to nourish the brain." When Chi is led to the head, it stays at the the Upper Dan Tien (center of forehead). The Upper Dan Tien is the residence of Shen. Chi and Shen are mutually related. When your Shen is weak, your Chi is weak, and your body will degenerate rapidly. Shen is the headquarters of Chi. Likewise, Chi supports the Shen, energizing it and keeping it sharp, clear, and strong. If the Chi in your body is weak, your Shen will also be weak.

2-3. Chi Kung Training Theory

In Chi Kung training, you must understand the principle behind everything you are doing. The principle is the root of your practice, and it

---

* Before birth you have no Chi of your own, but rather you use your mother's Chi. When you are born, you start creating Chi from the Original Jieng which you received from your parents. This Chi is called Pre-birth Chi, as well as Original Chi. It is also called Pre-Heaven Chi (Shian Tian Chi) because it comes from the Original Jieng which you received before you saw the heavens (which here means sky), i.e. before your birth.

is this root which brings forth the results you want. The root gives life, while the branches and flowers (results) give only temporary beauty. If you keep the root, you can regrow. If you have just branches and flowers, they will die in a short time.

Every Chi Kung form or practice has its special purpose and theory. If you do not know the purpose and theory, you have lost the root (meaning) of the practice. Therefore, as a Chi Kung practitioner, you must continue to ponder and practice until you understand the root of every set or form.

Before you start training, you must first understand that all of the training originates in your mind. You must have a clear idea of what you are doing, and your mind must be cal, centered, and balanced. This also implies that your feeling, sensing, and judgement must be objective and accurate. This requires emotional balance and a clear mind. This takes a lot of hard work, but once you have reached this level, you will have built the root of your physical training, and your Yi will be able to lead your Chi throughout your physical body.

As mentioned previously, Chi Kung training includes five important elements: regulating the body, regulating the breath, regulating the Yi (mind), regulating the Chi, and regulating the Shen (spirit). These are the foundation of successful Chi Kung practice. Without this foundation, your understanding of Chi Kung and your practice will remain superficial.

1. Regulating the Body

Regulating the Body is called "Tyau Shenn" in Chinese. This means to adjust your body until it is in the most comfortable and relaxed state. This implies that your body must be centered and balanced. If it is not, you will be tense and uneasy, and this will affect the judgement of your Yi and the circulation of your Chi. In Chinese medical society it is said: "(When) shape (body's posture) is not correct, then the Chi will not be smooth. (When) the Chi is not smooth, the Yi (mind) will not be peaceful. (When) the Yi is not peaceful, then the Chi is disordered."(1) You should understand that the relaxation of your body originates with your Yi. Therefore, before you can relax your body, you must first relax or regulate your mind (Yi). This is called "Shenn Hsin Pyng Herng", which means "Body and heart (mind) balanced." The body and the mind are mutually related. A relaxed and balanced body helps your Yi to relax and concentrate. When your Yi is at peace and can judge things accurately, your body will be centered, balanced, and relaxed.

Relaxation

Relaxation is one of the major keys to success in Chi Kung. You should remember that **ONLY WHEN YOU ARE RELAXED WILL ALL YOUR MUSCLES BE RELAXED, AND YOUR CHI CHANNELS OPEN.** In order to be relaxed, your Yi must first be relaxed and calm. When this Yi coordinates with your breathing, your body will be able to relax.

In Chi Kung practice, there are three levels of relaxation. The first level is the external physical relaxation, or postural relaxation. This is a very

---

(1).　"形不正則氣不順，氣不順則意不寧，意不寧則氣散亂。"

superficial level, and almost anyone can reach it. It consists of adopting a comfortable stance and avoiding unnecessary strain in how you stand and move. The second level is the relaxation of the muscles and tendons. To do this your Yi must be directed deep into the muscles and tendons. This relaxation will help open your Chi channels, and will allow the Chi to sink and accumulate in the Dan Tien..

The final stage is the relaxation which reaches the internal organs and the bone marrow. Remember, **ONLY IF YOU CAN RELAX DEEP INTO YOUR BODY WILL YOUR MIND BE ABLE TO LEAD THE CHI THERE.** Only at this stage will the Chi be able to reach everywhere. Then you will feel transparent — as if your whole body had disappeared. If you can reach this level of relaxation, you will be able to communicate with your organs and use Chi Kung to adjust or regulate the Chi disorders which are giving you problems. Not only that, you will be able to protect your organs more effectively, and therefore slow down their degeneration.

Rooting

In all Chi Kung practice, it is very important to be rooted. Being rooted means to be stable and in firm contact with the ground. If you want to push a car, you have to be rooted so the force you exert into the car will be balanced by a force into the ground. If you are not rooted, when you push the car you will only push yourself away, and not move the car. Your root is made up of your body's root, center, and balance.

Before you can develop your root, you must first relax and let your body "settle". As you relax, the tension in the various parts of your body will disolve, and you will find a comfortable way to stand. You will stop fighting the ground to keep your body up, and will learn to rely on your body's structure to support itself. This lets the muscles relax even more. Since your body isn't struggling to stand up, your Yi won't be pushing upward, and your body, mind, and Chi will all be able to sink. If you let dirty water sit quietly, the impurities will gradually settle down to the bottom, leaving the water above it clear. In the same way, if you relax your body enough to let it settle, your Chi will sink to your Dan Tien and the Bubbling Wells in your feet, and your mind will become clear. Then you can begin to develop your root.

To root your body you must imitate a tree and grow an invisible root under your feet. This will give you a firm root to keep you stable in your training. You should know that **YOUR ROOT MUST BE WIDE AS WELL AS DEEP.** Naturally, your Yi must grow first, because it is the Yi which leads the Chi. Your Yi must be able to lead the Chi to your feet, and be able to communicate with the ground. Only when your Yi can communicate with the ground will your Chi be able to grow beyond your feet and enter the ground to build the root. The Bubbling Well cavity is the gate which enables your Chi to communicate with the ground.

After you have gained your root, you must learn how to keep your center. A stable center will make your Chi develop evenly and uniformly. If you lose this center, your Chi will not be led evenly. In order to keep your body centered, you must first center your Yi, and then match your body to it. Only under these conditions will the Chi Kung forms you practice have their root. Your mental and physical center is the key which enables you to lead your Chi beyond your body.

Balance is the product of rooting and centering. Balance includes balancing the Chi and the physical body. It does not matter which aspect of balance you are dealing with, first you must balance your Yi, and only then can you balance your Chi and your physical body. If your Yi is balanced, it can help you to make accurate judgements, and therefore to correct the path of the Chi flow.

Rooting includes rooting not just the body, but also the form or movement. The root of any form or movement is found in its purpose or principle. For example, in certain Chi Kung exercises you want to lead the Chi to your palms. In order to do this, you must image* that you are pushing an object forward while keeping your muscles relaxed. In this exercise, your elbows must be down to build the sense of root for the push. If you raise the elbows, you lose the sense of "intention" of the movement, because the push would be ineffective if you were pushing something for real. Since the intention or purpose of the movement is its reason for being, you now have a purposeless movement, and you have no reason to lead Chi in any particular way. Therefore, in this case, the elbow is the root of the movement.

2. Regulating the Breath

Regulating breathing means to regulate your breath until it is calm, smooth, and peaceful. Only when you have reached this point will you be able to make the breathing deep, slender, long, and soft, which is required for successful Chi Kung practice.

Breathing is affected by your emotions. For example, when you are angry, you exhale more strongly than you inhale. When you are sad, you inhale more strongly than you exhale. When your mind is peaceful and calm, your inhalation and exhalation are relatively equal. In order to keep your breathing calm, peaceful, and steady, your mind and emotions must first be calm and neutral. Therefore, in order to regulate your breathing, you must first regulate your mind.

The other side of the coin is that you can use your breathing to control your Yi. When your breathing is uniform, it is as if you were hypnotizing your Yi, which helps to calm it. From this, you can see that Yi and breathing are interdependent, and that they cooperate with each other. Deep and calm breathing relaxes you and keeps your mind clear. It fills your lungs with plenty of air, so that your brain and entire body have an adequate supply of oxygen. In addition, deep and complete breathing enables the diaphragm to move up and down, which massages and stimulates the internal organs. For this reason, deep breathing exercises are also called "internal organ exercises."

Deep and complete breathing does not mean that you inhale and exhale to the maximum. This would cause the lungs and the surrounding muscles to tense up, which in turn would keep the air from circulating freely, and hinder the absorption of oxygen. Without enough oxygen, your mind becomes scattered, and the rest of your body tenses up. In correct breathing, you inhale and exhale to about 70% or 80% of capacity, so that your lungs stay relaxed.

You can conduct an easy expeiment. Inhale deeply so that your lungs are completely full, and time how long you can hold your breath. Then try

---

* The verb "image" used here means to mentally create something that you treat as if it were real. If you image that you are pushing something heavy, you have to adjust your posture exactly as if you were in fact pushing something heavy. You must "feel" its weight, the resistance as you exert force against it, and the force and counterforce in your legs. If you mentally treat your actions as real, your body will too, and the Chi will automatically move appropriately for those actions. If you only "pretend" or "imagine" that you are pushing something heavy, your mind and body will not treat your actions as real, and the Chi will not move strongly or clearly.

inhaling to only about 70% of your capacity, and see how long you can hold your breath. You will find that with the latter method you can last much longer than with the first one. This is simply because the lungs and the surrounding muscles are relaxed. When they are relaxed, the rest of your body and your mind can also relax, which significantly decreases your need for oxygen. Therefore, when you regulate your breathing, the first priority is to keep your lungs relaxed and calm.

When training, your mind must first be calm so that your breathing can be regulated. When the breathing is regulated, your mind is able to reach a higher level of calmness. This calmness can again help you to regulate the breathing, until your mind is deep. After you have trained for a long time, your breathing will be full and slender, and your mind will be very clear. It is said: "Hsin Shyi Shiang Yi", which means "Heart (mind) and breathing (are) mutually dependent." When you reach this meditative state, your heartbeat slows down, and your mind is very clear: you have entered the sphere of real meditation.

An Ancient Taoist named Li, Ching-Yen said: "Regulating breathing means to regulate the real breathing until (you) stop."(2) This means that correct regulating means not regulating. In other words, although you start by consciously regulating your breath, you must get to the point where the regulating happens naturally, and you no longer have to think about it. When you breathe, if you concentrate your mind on your breathing, then it is not true regulating, because the Chi in your lungs will become stagnant. When you reach the level of true regulating, no regulating is necessary, and you can use your mind efficiently to lead the Chi. Remember **WHEREVER THE YI IS, THERE IS THE CHI. IF THE YI STOPS IN ONE SPOT, THE CHI WILL BE STAGNANT. IT IS THE YI WHICH LEADS THE CHI AND MAKES IT MOVE.** Therefore, when you are in a state of correct breath regulation, your mind is free. There is no sound, stagnation, urgency, or hesitation, and you can finally be calm and peaceful.

You can see that when the breath is regulated correctly, the Chi will also be regulated. They are mutually related and cannot be separated. This idea is explained frequently in Taoist literature. The Taoist Kuan Chen Tzu said: "One exhale, the Earth Chi rises; one inhale, the Heaven Chi descends; real man's (meaning one who has attained the real Tao) repeated breathing at the navel, then my real Chi is naturally connected."(3) This says that when you breathe you should move your abdomen, as if you were breathing from your navel. The earth Chi is the negative (Yin) energy from your kidneys, and the sky Chi is the positive (Yang) energy which comes from the food you eat and the air you breathe. When you breathe from the navel, these two Chi's will connect and combine. Some people think that they know what Chi is, but they really don't. Once you connect the two Chi's, you will know what the "real" Chi is, and you may become a "real" man, which means to attain the Tao.

The Taoist book *Chain Tao Jing Yen* (Sing (of the) Tao (with) Real

---

(2).　"調息要調無息息"

(3).　廣成子曰："一呼則地氣上升，一吸則天氣下降，人之反覆呼吸於蒂，則我之真炁自然相接。"

Words) says: "One exhale one inhale to communicate Chi's function, one movement one calmness is the same as (is the source of) creation and variation."(4) The first part of this statement again implies that the functioning of Chi is connected with the breathing. The second part of this sentence means that all creation and variation come from the interaction of movement (Yang) and calmness (Yin). *Huang Ting Ching* (Yellow Yard Classic) says: "Breathe Original Chi to seek immortality."(5) In China, the traditional Taoists wore yellow robes, and they meditated in a "yard" or hall. This sentence means that in order to reach the goal of immortality, you must seek to find and understand the Original Chi which comes from the Dan Tien through correct breathing.

Moreover, the Taoist Wu Jen Zen said: "Use the post-birth breathing to look for the real person's (i.e. the immortal's) breathing place."(6) In this sentence, it is clear that in order to locate the immortal breathing place (the Dan Tien), you must rely on and know how to regulate your post-birth, or natural, breathing. Through regulating your post-birth breathing, you will gradually be able to locate the residence of the Chi (the Dan Tien), and eventually you will be able to use your Dan Tien to breath like the immortal Taoists. Finally, in the Taoist song *Ling Yuen Da Tao Gar* (The Great Taoist Song of the Spirit's Origin) it is said: "The Originals (Original Jieng, Chi, and Shen) are internally transported peacefully, so that you can become real (immortal); (if you) depend (only) on external breathing (you) will not reach the end (goal)."(7) From this song, you can see that internal breathing (breathing at the Dan Tien) is the key to training your three treasures and finally reaching immortality. However, you must first know how to regulate your external breathing correctly.

From the above, you can see the importance of breathing. There are eight key words for air breathing which a Chi Kung practitioner should follow during his exercise. Once you understand them you will be able to substantially shorten the time needed to reach your Chi Kung goals. These eight key words are: 1. Calm (Jing); 2. Slender (Shyi); 3. Deep (Shenn); 4. Long (Charng); 5. Continuous (Iou); 6. Uniform (Yun); 7. Slow (Hoan); and 8. Soft (Mian). These key words are self-explanatory, and with a little thought you should be able to understand them.

3. Regulating the Yi (Mind)

It is said in Taoist society that: "(When) large Tao is taught, first stop thought; when thought is not stopped, (the lessons are) in vain."(8) This

---

(4).　唱道真言曰：〝一呼一吸通乎炁機，一動一靜同乎造化。〞

(5).　黃庭經曰：〝呼吸元氣以求仙。〞

(6).　伍真人曰：〝用後天之呼吸，尋真人呼吸處。〞

(7).　靈源大道歌曰：〝元和內運即成真，呼吸外求終末了。〞

(8).　〝大道教人先止念，念頭不住亦徒然〞

means that when you first practice Chi Kung, the most difficult training is to stop your thinking. The final goal for your mind is "the thought of no thought."(9) Your mind does not think of the past, the present, or the future. Your mind is completely separated from influences of the present such as worry, happiness, and sadness. Then your mind can be calm and steady, and can finally gain peace. Only when you are in the state of "the thought of no thought" will you be relaxed and able to sense calmly and accurately.

Regulating your mind means using your consciousness to stop the activity in your mind in order to set it free from the bondage of ideas, emotion, and conscious thought. When you reach this level, your mind will be calm, peaceful, empty, and light. Then your mind has really reached the goal of relaxation. Only when you reach this stage will you be able to relax deep into your marrow and internal organs. Only then will your mind be clear enough to see (feel) the internal Chi circulation and communicate with your Chi and organs. In Taoist society it is called "Nei Shyh Kung Fu", which means the Kung Fu of internal vision.

When you reach this real relaxation, you may be able to sense the different elements which make up your body: solid matter, liquids, gases, energy, and spirit. You may even be able to see or feel the different colors that are associated with your five organs — green (liver), white (lungs), black (kidneys), yellow (spleen), and red (heart).

Once your mind is relaxed and regulated and you can sense your internal organs, you may decide to study the five element theory. This is a very profound subject, and it is sometimes interpreted differently by Oriental Physicians and Chi Kung practitioners. When understood properly, it can give you a method of analyzing the interrelationships between your organs, and help you devise ways to correct imbalances.

For example, the lungs correspond to the element Metal, and the heart to the element Fire. Metal (the lungs) can be used to adjust the heat of the Fire (the heart), because metal can take a large quantity of heat away from fire, (and thus cool down the heart). When you feel uneasy or have heartburn (excess fire in the heart), you may use deep breathing to calm down the uneasy emotions or cool off the heartburn.

Naturally, it will take a lot of practice to reach this level. In the beginning, you should not have any ideas or intentions, because they will make it harder for your mind to relax and empty itself of thoughts. Once you are in a state of "no thought", place your attention on your Dan Tien. It is said "Yi Shoou Dan Tien", which means "The Mind is kept on the Dan Tien." The Dan Tien is the origin and residence of your Chi. Your mind can build up the Chi here (start the fire, Chii For), then lead the Chi anywhere you wish, and finally lead the Chi back to its residence. When your mind is on the Dan Tien, your Chi will always have a root. When you keep this root, your Chi will be strong and full, and it will go where you want it to. You can see that when you practice Chi Kung, your mind cannot be completely empty and relaxed. You must find the firmness within the relaxation, then you can reach your goal.

In Chi Kung training, it is said: "Use your Yi (mind) to **LEAD** your Chi" (Yii Yi Yiin Chi). Notice the word **LEAD**. Chi behaves like water—it cannot be pushed, but it can be led. When Chi is led, it will flow smoothly and without stagnation. When it is pushed, it will flood and enter the

(9).　"無念之念"

wrog paths. Remember, wherever your Yi goes first, the Chi will naturally follow. For example, if you intend to lift an object, this intention is your Yi. This Yi will lead the Chi to the arms to energize the physical muscles, and then the object can be lifted.

It is said: "Your Yi cannot be on your Chi. Once your Yi is on your Chi, the Chi is stagnant." When you want to walk from one spot to another, you must first mobilize your intention and direct it to the goal, then your body will follow. The mind must always be ahead of the body. If your mind stays on your body, you will not be able to move.

In Chi Kung training, the first thing is to know what Chi is. If you do not know what Chi is, how will you be able to lead it? Once you know what Chi is and experience it, then your Yi will have something to lead. The next thing in Chi Kung training is knowing how your Yi communicates with your Chi. That means that your Yi should be able to sense and feel the Chi flow and understand how strong and smooth it is. In Tai Chi Chi Kung society, it is commonly said that your Yi must "listen" to your Chi and "understand" it. Listen means to pay careful attention to what you sense and feel. The more you pay attention, the better you will be able to understand. Only after you understand the Chi situation will your Yi be able to set up the strategy. In Chi Kung your mind or Yi must generate the idea (visualize your intention), which is like an order to your Chi to complete a certain mission.

The more your Yi communicates with your Chi, the more efficiently the Chi can be led. For this reason, as a Chi Kung beginner, you must first learn about Yi and Chi, and also learn how to help them communicate efficiently. Yi is the key in Chi Kung practice. Without this Yi you will not be able to lead your Chi, let alone build up the strength of the Chi or circulate it throughout your entire body.

Remember **WHEN THE YI IS STRONG, THE CHI IS STRONG, AND WHEN THE YI IS WEAK, THE CHI IS WEAK.** Therefore, the first step of Chi Kung training is to develop your Yi. The first secret of a strong Yi is **CALMNESS.** When you are calm, you can see things clearly and not be disturbed by surrounding distractions. With your mind calm, you will be able to concentrate.

Confucius said: "First you must be calm, then your mind can be steady. Once your mind is steady, then you are at peace. Only when you are at peace are you able to think and finally gain."(10) This procedure is also applied in meditation or Chi Kung exercise: **Calm** first, then **Steady, Peace, Think,** and finally **Gain.** That means when you practice Chi Kung, first you must learn to be calm (emotional calmness). Once calm, you will be able to see what you want and firm your mind (steady). This firm and steady mind is your intention or Yi (it is how your Yi is generated). Only after you know what you really want will your mind gain peace and be able to relax (emotional and physical relaxation). After you have reached this step, you must then concentrate or think in order to execute your intention. Under this thoughtful and concentrated mind, your Chi will follow and you will be able to gain what you wish.

---

(10). 孔子曰："先靜爾后有定，定爾后能安，安爾后能慮，慮爾后能得。"

4. Regulating the Chi

Before you can regulate your Chi, you must first regulate your body, breath, and mind. If you compare your body to a battlefield, then your mind is like the general who generates ideas and controls the situation, and your breathing is the strategy. Your Chi is like the soldiers who are led to various places on the battlefield. All four elements are necessary, and all four must be coordinated with each other if you are to win the war against sickness and aging.

If you want to arrange your soldiers most effectively for battle, you must know which area of the battlefield is most important, and where you are weakest (where your Chi is deficient) and need to send reinforcements. If you have more soldiers than you need in one area (excessive Chi), then you can send them somewhere else where the ranks are thin. As a general, you must also know how many soldiers are available for the battle, and how many you will need for protecting yourself and your headquarters. To be successful, not only do you need good strategy (breathing), but you also need to communicate and understand the situation effectively with your troops, or all of your strategy will be in vain. When your Yi (the general) knows how to regulate the body (knows the battlefield), how to regulate the breathing (set up the strategy), and how to effectively regulate the Chi (direct your soldiers), you will be able to reach the final goal of Chi Kung training.

In order to regulate your Chi so that it moves smoothly in the correct paths, you need more than just efficient Yi-Chi communication. You also need to know how to generate the Chi. If you do not have enough Chi in your body, how can you regulate it? In a battle, if you do not have enough soldiers to set up your strategy, you have already lost.

When you practice Chi Kung, you must first train to make your Chi flow naturally and smoothly. There are some Chi Kung exercises in which you intentionally hold your Yi, and thus Chi, in a specific area. As a beginner, however, you should first learn how to make the Chi flow smoothly instead of building a Chi dam, which is commonly done in external martial Chi Kung training.

In order to make Chi flow naturally and smoothly, your Yi must first be relaxed. Only when your Yi is relaxed will your body be relaxed and the Chi channels open for the Chi to circulate. Then you must coordinate your Chi flow with your breathing. Breathing regularly and calmly will make your Yi calm, and allow your body to relax.

5. Regulating the Shen (Spirit)

There is one thing that is more important than anything else in a battle, and that is fighting spirit. You may have the best general, who knows the battlefield well and is also an expert strategist, but if his soldiers do not have a high fighting spirit (morale), he might still lose. Remember, **SPIRIT IS THE CENTER AND ROOT OF A FIGHT.** When you keep this center, one soldier can be equal to ten soldiers. When his spirit is high, a soldier will obey his orders accurately and willingly, and his general will be able to control the situation efficiently. In a battle, in order for a soldier to have this kind of morale, he must know why he is fighting, how to fight, and what he can expect after the fight. Under these conditions, he will know what he is doing and why, and this understanding will raise up his spirit, strengthen his will, and increase his patience and endurance.

It is the same with Chi Kung training. In order to reach the final goal of Chi Kung exercise, you must have three fundamental spiritual roots: will, patience, and endurance. You must know why, how, and what. Only then will you be able to be sure of your target and know what you are doing.

Shen, which is the Chinese term for spirit, originates from Yi (the general). When Shen is strong, the Yi is firm. When the Yi is firm, Shen will be steady and calm. From this you can see that **SHEN IS THE MENTAL PART OF A SOLDIER. WHEN SHEN IS HIGH, THE CHI IS STRONG AND EASILY DIRECTED. WHEN THE CHI IS STRONG, SHEN IS ALSO STRONG.**

CHAPTER 3

SITTING EIGHT PIECES OF BROCADE

It has been nearly one thousand years since the Eight Pieces of Brocade were created. There are many versions, each one somewhat different from the others. However, it does not matter which version you are training, the basic principles and theory are the same, and the goal is consistent. Remember that the most important thing in the training is not the forms themselves, but rather the theory and principle of each form, which constitute its root. Once you understand these, you will be able to use your Yi (mind) to lead the Chi to circulate and bring you to health. Therefore, when you practice you should try to understand the poetry or the "secret words." They have been passed down for hundreds of years, and are the root of the practice. Because of cultural and language differences, it is very difficult to translate into English all of the meaning of the Chinese. We will try to keep as close as possible to the Chinese, and hope that you are able to get not just the meaning, but also the taste of the original. Sometimes, words that are not in the original will be added in parentheses to clarify the meaning. Each section of poetry will be discussed so that it is as clear as possible.

As the first chapter explains, The Eight Pieces of Brocade is a Wai Dan (External Elixir) exercise. It includes both types of Wai Dan Chi Kung practice theory: not only does it build up Chi in the limbs and then allow this Chi to flow into the organs, but it also uses the motion of the limbs to move the muscles around the organs and increase the Chi circulation there.

There are two sets of The Eight Pieces of Brocade. One set is "sitting" and the other is "standing." The sitting set discussed in this chapter focuses on exercising the upper limbs, and benefits the six organs which are related to the six Chi channels in the arms. The sitting set is a good way to wake up in the morning, and it is usually practiced before noon. The sitting set is also good for people who are bedridden or cannot stand easily.

You may wonder about the number of repetitions directed for the different exercises. Chinese people consider 12 to be the number of a cycle; for example, 12 months comprise a year. Therefore, you will often see twelve or its multiples listed as the recommended numbers of repetitions. Square numbers such as 9, 16, 49, or 64 are also popular. Such numbers are only a guide, and you don't need to follow them precisely. If you have only a limited amount of time, and cannot do the recommended number of repetitions, simply use a smaller number. Do not, however, omit any of the exercises.

You may have noticed that in the discussion of the training theory and in the training instructions there is very little about coordinating your breathing with the movements. This is simply because the set was designed for the beginning Chi Kung practitioner. For the beginner, the most important element of the practice is relaxation. Only when you have mastered the set and learned how to regulate your body should you start to coordinate your breath with the movements. The general rule in breathing is that when you extend your limbs you exhale and lead the Chi to the extremities, and when you withdraw your limbs, you inhale and lead the Chi to your spine.

Sitting Eight Pieces of Brocade
First Piece: Bih Muh Jing Tzuoh (Close eyes and sit still)

閉目靜坐

Secret Words: Close eyes and sit with deep mind, (hands) hold firm, (mind is) calm, and think (concentrate on the) Shen (spirit).

閉目冥心坐，握固靜思神．

Practice: Sit with your legs crossed and concentrate on your solar plexus. Your head should feel as if it were suspended, and your chest loose and relaxed. The waist and spine are easy and comfortable. Hold your hands in your lap (Figure 3-1). Your mouth is closed and the teeth are touching slightly. Regulate your breathing so that it is smooth and uniform. Your mind is clear and pure. Condense your Yi (mind) and Shen (spirit) internally, until the Shen is peaceful and the Chi sinks. Your Yi is on the center Dan Tien (solar plexus). You should meditate at least 3-5 minutes.

Discussion: Three places are called Dan Tien (field of elixir): the forehead is called the Shang Dan Tien (Upper Dan Tien), the solar plexus is the Jong Dan Tien (Middle Dan Tien), and the abdomen is the Shiah Dan Tien (Lower Dan Tien). The Upper Dan Tien is the residence of Shen (spirit), where the Chi can be gathered and then directed by the Shen to circulate throughout the entire body. The Middle Dan Tien is the center where the Post-birth Chi accumulates. Post-birth Chi is obtained mainly from food and air. When Chi in the Middle Dan Tien is stimulated and full, the body is energized. The mind, however, although stimulated to a higher state, is scattered, and you will be troubled by heartburn. The Lower Dan Tien, which is the original source of human life, is the residence of Pre-birth Chi.

This exercise will extinguish any fire in your Middle Dan Tien so that you can concentrate and calm your mind. Before you start any Chi Kung exercise, you must first be calm. Closing your eyes will keep you from seeing anything distracting which is happening around you, and help you to calm down. You must train yourself to meditate with a deep mind. When you practice, hold your hands in front of your abdomen. Holding them together will help you to keep your mind centered and firm. If you wish, you may regulate your breath for a minute to start calming your mind, but then let go of the regulating and allow your mind to be calm and deep. Concentrate on your middle Dan Tien to calm down the Post-birth fire Chi. When the fire is gone, place your concentrated mind on your Shen, which is located in the upper Dan Tien, to increase your energy level.

In China, concentration is called "Jiuh Jieng Huey Shen" (gathering your Jieng and meeting with Shen). Jieng here does not mean semen or sperm, but rather something which is refined. Here it means the refined and concentrated mind. When the mind meets with Shen (spirit), the Shen will be raised. Whenever your Shen is raised, you will be able to increase the depth of your concentration.

Second Piece: Shoou Baw Kuen Luen (Hands hold Kuen Luen)

手把崑崙

Secret Words: Knock the teeth thirty-six (times), two hands hold Kuen Luen (head).

叩齒三十六，兩手把崑崙．

Practice: First tap your teeth together 36 times. If there is any saliva generated, swallow it. Then fold your hands together and hold the back of your head (Figure 3-2). Push your head and body backward while pulling your hands forward. Inhale when tensing, exhale when relaxing. Repeat 9 times.

Discussion: There are two major purposes for tapping the teeth together. One purpose is to stimulate the Chi in the gums to strengthen the roots of the teeth. In ancient times, dentists and technology were not as common or advanced as today, and you had to take care of your teeth by yourself. Tapping your teeth together strengthens the roots and helps prevent decay. The other purpose is to clear and waken the mind. When you tap,

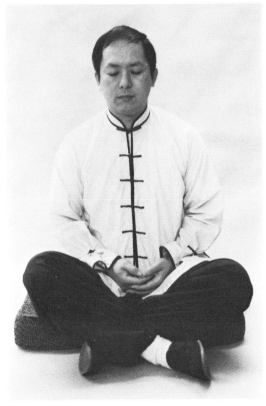

Figure 3-1.

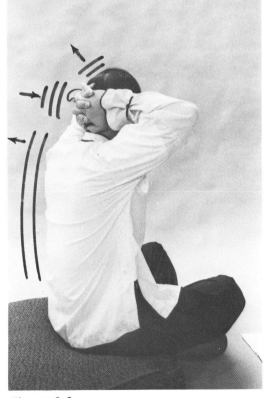

Figure 3-2.

the vibrations resonate in your brain cavity and stimulate the brain. This will clear the mind.

Kuen Luen mountain is one of the highest mountains in China. Here it means your head, which is the highest part of your body. When you push your head backward while pulling your hands forward, also push out your whole back. This will straighten the spine. In addition, this exercise tenses and then relaxes the back muscles, which will increase the Chi circulation there and in the Governing Vessel. This exercise will also strengthen the spine and prevent backache. When you are doing this piece, your breathing should be coordinated with the movement to help the lungs compress and expand. This will release tension in the lungs and increase lung capacity.

Third Piece: Kow Jyi Yuh Jeen (Knock and beat the Jade Pillow)

叩擊玉枕

Secret Words: Left right beat the heavenly drum, resounding twenty-four times.

左右鳴天鼓，二十四度聞。

Practice: Continue from the last piece. Cover your ears with your palms, with the middle fingers on the Jade Pillow cavity area (under the external occipital protuberance)(Figure 3-3). Put your index fingers on the middle fingers, and snap them down to hit your head (Figure 3-4). This will generate a drumming sound in the brain cavity. This exercise is commonly called "Ming Tian Guu", which means "sound the heavenly drum." Hit 24 times in an even, steady beat. You may hit with both fingers at the same time, or else alternate the fingers.

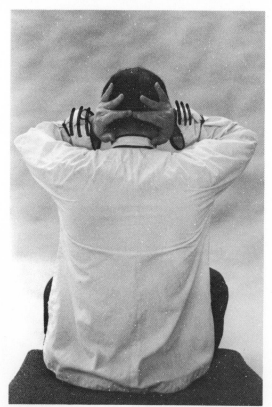

Figure 3-3.

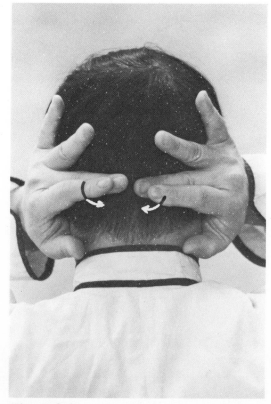

Figure 3-4.

Discussion: The Jade Pillow (Yuh Jeen) is the name of a cavity located on the back of your head under the protruding ridge of bone. The heavenly drum means the head.

When you do this exercise, do not let your ring and pinky fingers touch your head, for this will muffle the sound. Concentrate on the sound, and let every beat bring your attention more fully to the vibrations in your skull and brain. Beating the drum clears the mind. When you are finished and take your hands off your ears, you will feel like you just woke up, and everything will seem clear.

Fourth Piece: Joan Tour Pyn Pyn or Wei Bae Tian Juh (Turn the head repeatedly, or Lightly swing the sky post)

轉頭頻頻（微擺天柱）

Secret Words: Lightly turn (the head) to loosen up the Tian Juh (sky post, i.e. neck). Red dragon (the tongue) stirs the liquid saliva, drum rinse thirty-six (times), saliva liquid fills the entire mouth, one mouthful divided into three swallows, use Yi to send (it) to the belly wheel (navel).

微擺撼天柱，赤龍攪水津，鼓漱三十六，津液滿口生，一口分三咽，以意送臍輪。

Practice: Continue from the last piece, move your hands down and place them in your lap, palms facing up comfortably. Keeping your shoulders still, turn your head to the left and then the right 24 times (Figure 3-5). After this, move your tongue around inside your mouth to generate saliva (Figures 3-6), then move the saliva around to rinse your mouth 36 times, which will also generate more saliva. Swallow this saliva in three gulps. Every time you swallow, use your Yi to send the saliva down to the navel.

Discussion: The head is considered the heavens, and the top of the head is called Tian Ling Gay (Heavenly Cover). The neck, which is supported by the two major muscles on the back of the neck, is thus called the Tian Juh, which means the post which supports the heavens. The Chinese word translated here as "loosen up" has the feeling of shaking something to let everything settle back into place. Eight of the fourteen Chi channels pass through the neck. As you turn your head back and forth, the neck muscles alternately stretch and relax, which clears the Chi channels as well as loosens up the muscles. This prevents the headache which is caused by stagnation of Chi in the head.

According to the Taoists, saliva is the water which is able to put out the fire in the body. For example, when you have a sore throat or heartburn, saliva will ease the pain and help you recover. Saliva is a natural product which is being constantly generated, and it will help you whenever it is needed. When the supply of saliva stops, it is a sign that your body is too positive, and you are about to become ill.

The Red Dragon refers to the tongue. Move your tongue around in your mouth to generate saliva, and then move the saliva around, pushing the cheeks out tight like a drum (drum rinse) to rinse your mouth (Figure 3-7). Swallowing the saliva will help to put out the fire of excess energy in the heart.

When you swallow, use your mind to lead the saliva down to the lower abdomen. Of course, the saliva doesn't really go that far, but if you act as

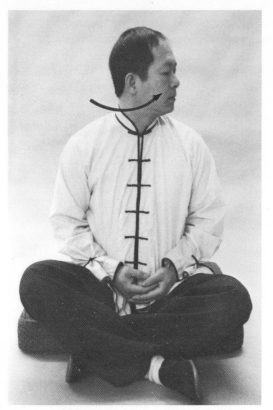

Figure 3-5

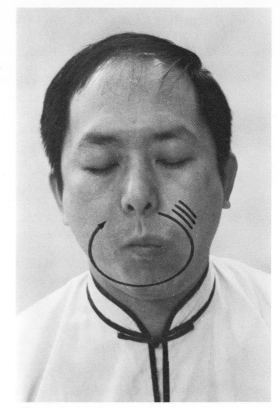

Figure 3-6.

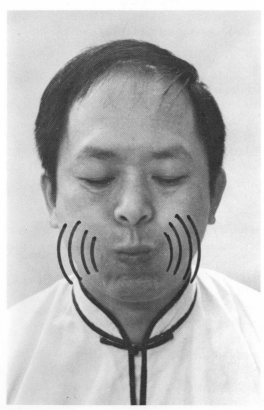

Figure 3-7.

if you were swallowing the saliva all the way down to your abdomen, you should be able to feel the energy from the saliva sinking to your Dan Tien.

The Chyi Luen, or "Belly Wheel", is a term which the Taoists commonly use for the navel. The Taoists, like the Buddhists, believe that people die and are reborn repeatedly in cycles that that move like a great wheel. The abdomen, specifically the navel area, is strongly involved in this reincarnation.

When the text says to bring the saliva to the belly wheel, it actually means the Dan Tien. The Eight Pieces of Brocade is a very simple Chi Kung set which was designed for the common people. These people would have little or no knowledge of internal things, and would not know what the Dan Tien is. The clearest and easiest way was to simply tell them to concentrate on the belly button. Everybody knows where that is, and it is close enough to the Dan Tien to be effective.

Fifth Piece: Tuei Mo Shenn Yu or Shoou Mo Jieng Men (Push and massage Shenn Yu, or Hands massage the Essence Door).

推摩腎俞（手摩精門）

Secret Words: Seal the breath and rub hands (until) hot, massage the rear Essence Door (on your) back, end this one mouthful of breath, think (image) the fire is burning the belly wheel.

閉氣搓手熱，背摩後精門，盡此一口
氣，想火燒臍輪。

Practice: Continue from the last piece. Inhale through your nose and lead the air to the middle Dan Tien (solar plexus), and hold the breath gently. Rub your hands together until they are warm (Figure 3-8). Then place your palms on the Shenn Yu cavity (kidneys), and press in as you massage with a circular motion 24 times (Figure 3-9). If you cannot hold your breath comfortably while you massage 24 times, don't strain. Only massage 12 times, or however many is comfortable for you, then exhale. Then inhale again, rub your hands, and repeat. When you massage, unite your Yi and Chi, and concentrate your Yi on the navel or Dan Tien. This concentration will make the abdomen get warm, or even hot. When you are finished with the massaging, sit quietly with your hands in your lap and feel the energy from your kidneys burning inside your navel or Dan Tien.

Discussion: Shenn Yu (Kidney Affirmative), which is also called Jieng Men (Essence Door), is the name of a cavity located in the kidney area. There are two of these cavities, one over each kidney. The kidneys are considered the residence of Original Jieng (Yuan Jieng)(also called Pre-birth Jieng). When this Jieng is converted into Chi it is called Original Chi (Yuan Chi), and it resides in the lower Dan Tien. It is believed that the Essence Door cavities are the door through which external Chi can reach the kidneys, and also the way by which the Original Chi generated by the kidneys can pass out of the body and be lost. It is also believed that the two kidneys are the root of the gonads (testicles or ovaries), which the Chinese call the external kidneys. When a person's kidneys are weak, his gonads will function poorly, and hormone production will be deficient. Such a person will be weak, his sexual vitality will be low, and his body will degenerate rapidly.

The person who practices Chinese meditation must learn how to keep

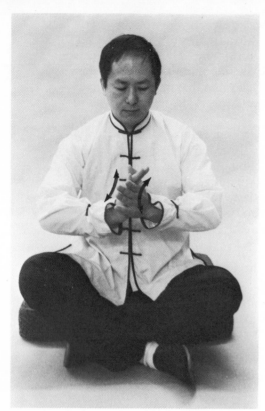

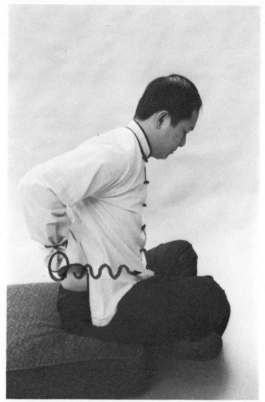

Figure 3-8.   Figure 3-9.

from losing his Jieng through his Essence Door. This is done through Dan Tien breathing, which takes Jieng from the kidneys and converts it to Chi, and stores this Chi in the Chi residence (Dan Tien). Therefore, instead of losing your Jieng, you gain Chi, and store it at the Dan Tien.

You must also learn how to use external Chi to warm the kidneys and stimulate the production of Original Chi or Jieng Chi, and how to store it in the Dan Tien so you can use it to improve your health. Therefore, in this piece you first rub your hands together to generate heat and Chi in your hands. When you rub your back with your warm hands, you pass Chi into the kidneys, which stimulates them to produce Original Chi. You don't want this Chi to pass out through the Essence Doors and disperse, so you bring it to the Dan Tien. This is done very simply by keeping your attention (Yi) on your Dan Tien. Since Chi follows Yi, the Chi you generate will automatically move where you are concentrating (Figure 3-9). It is said that the more Original Chi you have stored, the healthier and stronger you will be.

Sixth Piece: Shoou Joan Shuang Luen or Tzuoo Yow Luh Lu (Hands turns double wheel, or Left and right windlass)

手轉雙輪（左右轆轤）

Secret Words: Left and right windlasses turn, two feet lie comfortably extended.

左右轆轤轉，兩腳放舒伸。

Practice: Continue from the last piece. Extend your legs comfortably flat on the floor, with your arms at your sides, hands slightly forward and the palms facing down. The fingers are slightly curved and the elbows are bent. Move your arms in a vertical circle, with the motion coming from the shoulders, as if you were turning wheels with your hands (Figure 3-10). Rotate 9 times in one direction, then 9 times in the other direction.

Discussion: The motion is like turning wheels with both hands. Luh Lu means turning a wheel or rotating a windlass.

This piece is used mainly to increase Chi circulation in the six arm channels. You will feel the Chi generated from the circular shoulder motion reaching strongly out to the fingertips. Your legs are stretched out on the floor to open wide the other six Chi channels in the legs. Even though you are practicing circulating Chi in your hands, the Chi will also move out to your toes, because your body's natural instinct is to balance the Chi throughout your body.

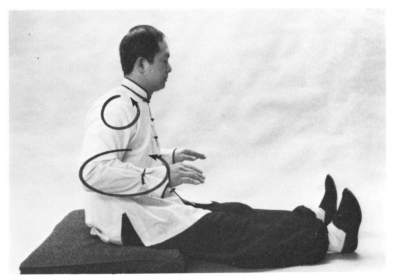

Figure 3-10

Seventh Piece: Tuo An Pan Tzwu (Lift; press; and hold the feet)

托按攀足

Secret Words: Interlock fingers of both (hands,) false lift, lower the head repeatedly to hold the feet.

义手雙虛托，低頭攀足頻 。

Practice: Continue from the last piece. Interlock your hands, and lift them above your head, palm up. Keep imaging that you are lifting and holding something up above your head (Figure 3-11). Stay there for about 3 seconds, then turn your palms down and touch the top of your head. Press your hands downward while you lift your head upward for about 3 seconds (Figure 3-12). Finally, separate your hands and bend forward, using your hands to pull back your toes (Figure 3-13). Keep your knees straight and stay in the position for about 3 seconds. Repeat the entire process 9 times.

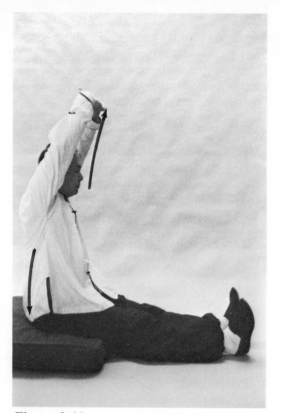

Figure 3-11.

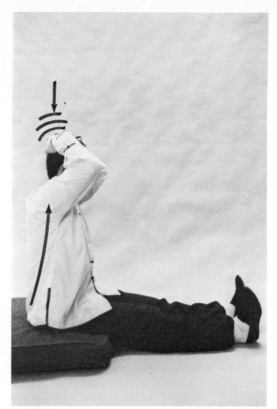

Figure 3-12.

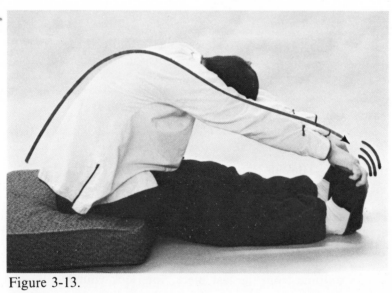

Figure 3-13.

Discussion: In this piece, you first interlock your hands and then push up above your head. Because there is nothing for you to push against, the Chinese call it a "false lift." When you push up over your head, you stretch the muscles in the front and back of your body. This stretching and relaxing movement helps to regulate the Sanjiao Chi channels. Sanjiao means "Triple Burner", and includes the upper, middle, and lower parts of your torso. The Upper Burner is located in the chest above the diaphragm, The Middle Burner is between the diaphragm and the navel, and the Lower Burner is located between the navel and the groin.

After you have loosened up the muscles, place your hands on the top of your head and press down. You balance this downward push with an upward push of your head. This upward push comes all the way from the floor. The Yi of pushing upward and downward will lead any stagnant Chi in the Sanjiao areas into the Small Circulation (the circular pathway through the Conception and Governing vessels).

Finally, hold your toes or feet and pull them back, letting your head hang down. This position stretches and slightly tenses the muscles in the back, and when you then sit up and raise your arms over your head, you release the tension. This alternately presses in on the kidneys, and then lets up, which increase the circulation of blood and Chi in the kidneys and keeps them healthy.

Another way to do the last part of this piece is to place your hands over your toes and press your middle fingers into the Bubbling Well cavities. Since these cavities are on the channels which connect with the kidneys, this method provides additional stimulation to the kidneys.

Eighth Piece: Jou Tian Mann Yunn (Entire sky slow transportation)

周天慢運

Secret Words: Wait until the mouth water arrives, again rinse again swallow the saliva, do this three times, swallow mouth water nine times, swallow noisily, (in) hundreds of vessels (Chi) adjusts uniformly (and) automatically, entire sky (body) slow transportation completed, think that fire is burning (your) entire body. Ancient name eight pieces of brocade, train after midnight and before noon, train diligently without ceasing, thousands of illnesses vanish into dust.

以候口水至，再漱再吞津，如此三度
畢，口水九次吞，咽下汨汨響，百脈
自調勻，周天慢運畢，想火遍燒身。
舊名八段錦，子後午前行，勤行無間
斷，萬病化為塵。

Practice: Cross your legs and place your hands in your lap. Close your eyes and sit calmly (Figure 3-14). When enough saliva accumulates, rinse and then swallow three times with an audible gulp. After you swallow, keep your attention on your navel or Dan Tien, and feel the Chi circulating smoothly throughout your body. When more saliva accumulates, rinse again and swallow three more times. Repeat once more, for a total of nine swallows. After this, relax and feel the Chi burning like a fire all over your body (Figure 3-15). This means that you should lead the Chi to your skin to form a protective shield around your

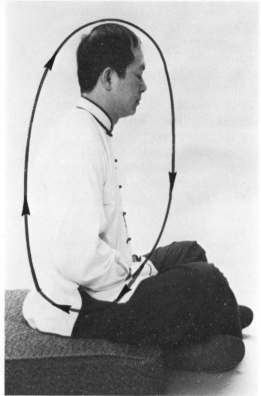

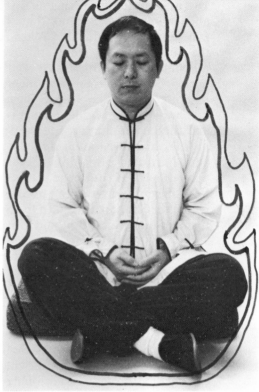

Figure 3-14.   Figure 3-15

body. After you have completed these eight pieces, sit quietly and breath evenly for about 3 minutes.

Discussion: When you have finished the preceding seven pieces, your body may be too positive, and you may have let Chi rise up in your body instead of settle down to the Dan Tien. Swallowing the saliva is a way to bring the Chi back down again. There are two ways to generate saliva. One is to move the tongue around in the mouth, and the other is to simply concentrate your mind on your mouth and let the saliva be generated spontaneously. Since this is the last piece, it is desirable to put out any fire you may have caused by the exercises. If you start moving your tongue around again, you may start generating more heat and fire. You simply want to calm down. That is why you use your Yi instead of your tongue to generate the saliva. In this piece, when you swallow, you do it "noisily." Bringing the saliva down with a big gulp helps to concentrate all of your attention, and makes it easier for you to relax.

You want the Chi you have accumulated in your Dan Tien to circulate throughout your body. When you sit quietly with your attention on your Dan Tien, the Chi will accumulate there. As it fills up the Dan Tien, it will become stimulated, gradually spreading out and filling the entire body. You will be able to feel the Chi moving throughout your body, clearing out obstructions in the channels, and automatically balancing itself. You may feel the Chi moving through what is called the Small Circulation (Figure 3-14), which is the circular path through the Governing Vessel on the back and the Conception Vessel down the center front of the body. When you are finished with the swallowing and the body is warm and full of Chi, image that the skin and the area around your body is full of fire. This image will bring Chi to the skin and build up the shield of Wei Chi (Guardian Chi) around the body.

CHAPTER 4

STANDING EIGHT PIECES OF BROCADE

The standing set of the Eight Pieces of Brocade is more popular than the sitting set, so there are more versions of it in the documents. You should not worry about which version is better or more accurate, because the basic principles are the same. It is more important that you really understand the root of the practice, and that you train patiently and perseveringly. Every piece has its own poem or song to explain the exercise and its purpose. The poems or songs have been passed down through generations, and form the root and foundation of each piece, so you should make a diligent effort to understand them. Whereas the sitting set emphasized the six Chi channels in the arms, the standing set works with all of the channels.

Standing Eight Pieces of Brocade
First Piece:
Double hands hold up the heavens to regulate the Sanjiao (Triple Burner); Sanjiao passes (Chi) freely and smoothly, illnesses disappear. Reverse hands to face the sky and raise both arms. Thrust out (straighten) your chest, straighten your waist (and) swing to both sides. Stand upright and be steady. Practice long, the body (becomes) strong (and you will feel) happy.

雙手托天理三焦，三焦通暢疾病消。
反手朝天振雙臂，挺胸直腰兩側搖。
立正姿勢要站穩，久練體牡樂陶陶。

Practice: Stand naturally with your feet parallel and shoulder width apart, and your hands at your sides. Close your eyes, calm down your mind, and breathe regularly (Figure 4-1). Open your eyes and look forward, continue breathing naturally and smoothly. Condense your Shen in your upper Dan Tien, and sink your Chi to the Lower Dan Tien. Then interlock your fingers and raise your hands above your head without bending your arms, and at the same time lift up your heels

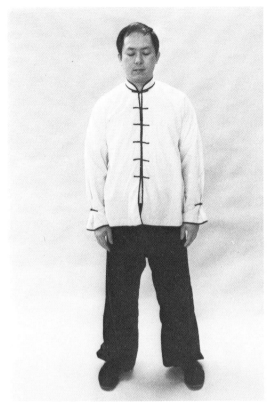

Figure 4-1.

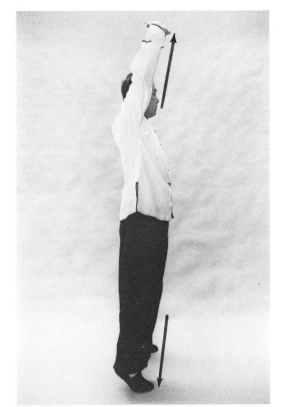

Figure 4-2.

(Figure 4-2). This is called "Double hands hold up the heavens" (Shuang Shoou Tuo Tian). Drop your heels, and tilt your body to the left and then to the right, and then stand up straight again (Figure 4-3). Lower your hands down in front of your body to complete one round. Do 24 repetitions.

Discussion: This set does not start with calm meditation, but since Chi Kung training is strongly related to your feelings, it is important for your mind to be calm and steady. It is a good idea to stand quietly for a while before you start, so that your mind can become calm.

From the poetry you can see that this piece works especially with the Sanjiao or Triple Burner. The three areas, or "burners", that are referred to are the area above the diaphragm, between the diaphragm and navel, and between the navel and the groin. The three burners are concerned respectively with respiration, digestion, and elimination. When you raise your hands over your head and tilt to either side you stretch the muscles of your trunk. When you let your arms down, the muscles loosen and relax, and the Chi can circulate unimpeded. Repeating the movement regulates the Chi circulation in your Sanjiao. When Sanjiao Chi circulation is smooth, the organs will be relaxed, and the organ Chi will be able to move and circulate freely. It is believed that disorders in the Sanjiao are the major cause of many organ Chi disorders. When Sanjiao Chi is regulated, the illness will disappear.

When you practice, you also lift up your heels. This helps you to generate an Yi of pushing up, which helps the Sanjiao Chi move up and down. When they say to "straighten your waist" they mean to keep your lower back straight.

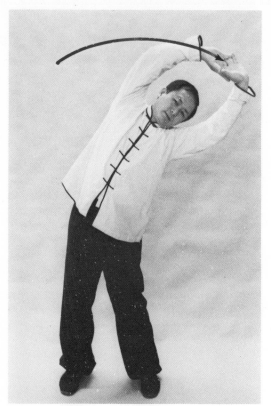

Figure 4-3.

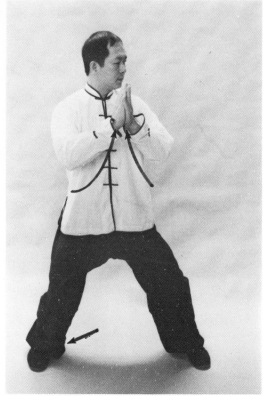

Figure 4-4.

Second Piece:

Left right open (bend) the bow like shooting a hawk, two arms strong and firm to strengthen kidneys and waist. Bend the elbow horizontal to the shoulder, (your mind) trying hard to pull. Hand arrow aims (at the target), use the eyes to stare. Left right shoot for twenty-four. Ride the horse and squat down to increase efficiency.

左右開弓似射雕，兩臂堅牢壯腎腰。
曲肘平肩努力拉，手箭對準用目瞄。
左右放射二十四，騎馬蹲襠効力高。

Practice: Step your right leg to the right and squat down in a horse stance. Relax your hands and lift them up to the chest area. Bring your palms together (Figure 4-4), then separate them with the right hand moving near the right nipple, while the left hand, changing into the "sword secret" or "single finger" hand form, extends to the left as if you were pulling a bow to shoot a hawk (Figure 4-5). Your eyes stare to your left at a very distant point. Then stand up and lower your hands, circle them up to the chest and repeat the same process to shoot to your right. Do 12 in either direction for a total of 24.

Discussion: This piece is used to strengthen the kidneys and the waist area. First you must squat down to firm your root as when you pull a strong bow. Without this root, you will not have a center, and you will not be able to pull your bow effectively. Make sure when you squat down that

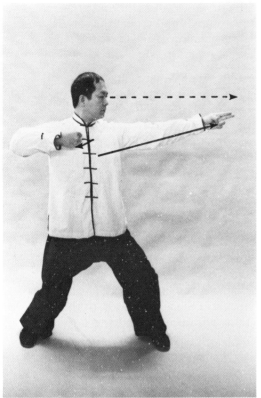

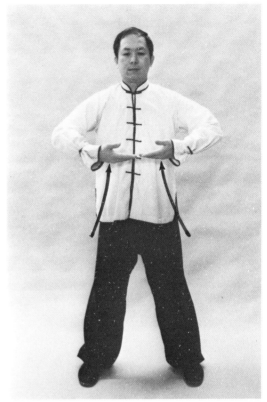

Figure 4-5

Figure 4-6.

you keep your back straight and tuck your buttocks under. This emphasizes the kidney area. When you are doing this, you not only strengthen the waist muscles but also increase the Chi circulation in the kidney area, which is in your back near your lowest ribs. Your rear elbow must be bent and the shoulders must be firm to stabilize the pulling of the bow. Concentrate your mind so that you really feel that you are drawing a very strong bow. This concentrated mind is the source of the Chi movement.

Third Piece:
To adjust and regulate the spleen and stomach, (you) must lift singly; spleen and stomach (gain) peace and harmony, sickness cured automatically. Lift arm and stiffen the palms, use the force to rock. Extend and develop the tendons and muscles, spleen and stomach comfortable. Right hand lifted high, left dropped down, left right extend and rock the tendons and channels alive.

調理脾胃須單舉，脾胃平和病自癒。
舉臂挺掌用力搖，抻撥筋肋脾胃舒。
右手高舉左下垂，左右抻搖筋絡活。

Practice: After you have completed the last piece, stand up and move your leg back so that the feet are parallel and shoulder width apart. Then move both hands to the front of your stomach with the palms facing up (Figure 4-6). Raise your left hand above your head and push upward, and at the same time lower your right hand palm down to your side and press down slightly (Figure 4-7). Then change your hands and repeat the same process. You should feel that both hands are pushing against resistance, but you must not tense your muscles. Do 24 repetitions.

Discussion: This piece works on the stomach. When you repeatedly raise one hand and lower the other, you loosen the muscles in the front of your body. When you "stiffen the palms", do not tense the muscles, but rather extend your force through the hands so that your arms stretch out all the way. This stimulates and strengthens the tendons and muscles. Reversing your arms repeatedly stretches and relaxes the body, "rocking" the tendons and Chi channels alive. This one-up-and-one-down muscle movement increases the Chi circulation in your stomach, spleen, and liver. If you wish, when you raise and stretch each hand you can also stretch the leg on the same side to increase the extension.

Fourth Piece:
Five weaknesses and seven injuries, wait and see later (they'll be gone); train long, exercise long, tendons and bones strong. Weakness injuries (from over-exertion) all because the internal organs (are) weak. Thrust out (straighten) the chest and twist the neck to take a good look to the rear. Hold the waist and hold up the chest, the body is upright. Especially effective in curing internal injury.

五勞七傷望後瞧，久練久作筋骨牢。
癆傷皆因內臟弱，挺胸扭脖後看好。
招腰捧胸身平立，專治內傷有功效。

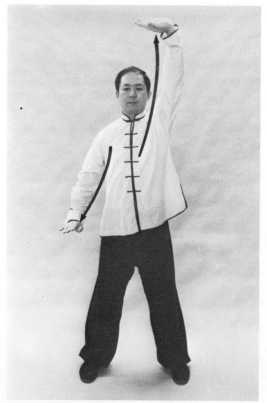

Figure 4-7.

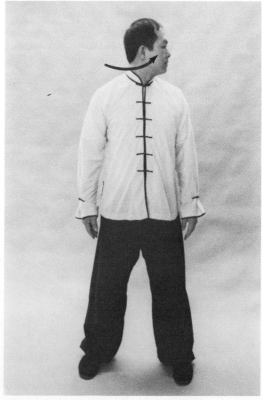

Figure 4-8.

-56-

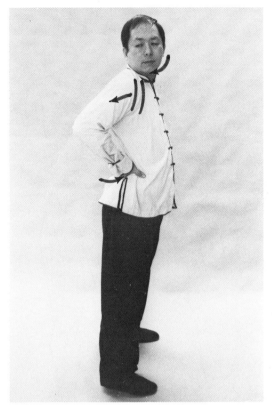

Figure 4-9.

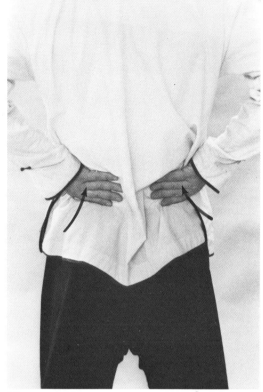

Figure 4-10

Practice: Stand easily and comfortably with both feet parallel as before, and your hands hanging down naturally at your sides. Lift your chest slightly from the inside so that your posture is straight, but be careful not to thrust your chest out. Turn your head to the left and look to the rear as you exhale (Figure 4-8), then return your head to the front as you inhale. Turn your head to the right and look to the rear as you exhale, then return your head to the front as you inhale. Turn twelve times in each direction, for a total of twenty-four. Your body should remain facing to the front. Do not turn it as you turn your head. Next, place your hands on your waist and turn your head 24 times as before (Figures 4-9 and 4-10). Finally, move both hands to your chest with the palms facing up, press your elbows and shoulders slightly forward, and repeat the head turning 24 times (Figure 4-11).

During all three parts, use your Yi to lead the Chi from the Dan Tien to your Bubbling Well (Yongquan cavity)(Figure 4-12) and Huiyin cavities (Figure 4-13) when you exhale and turn your head to either side, and then lead the Chi back to the Dan Tien as you inhale and return your head to the front.

Discussion: Five weaknesses refers to illnesses of the five Yin organs: heart, liver, spleen, lungs, and kidneys. The seven injuries refers to injuries caused by the seven emotions: happiness, anger, sorrow, joy, love, hate, and desire. According to Chinese medicine, you can become ill when your internal organs are weak, and emotional disturbance upsets them. For example, anger can cause the Chi in your liver to stagnate, which will affect the functioning of the organ. But your organs are not the

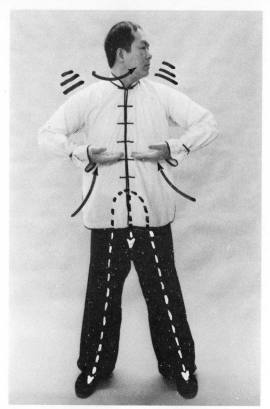

Figure 4-11.

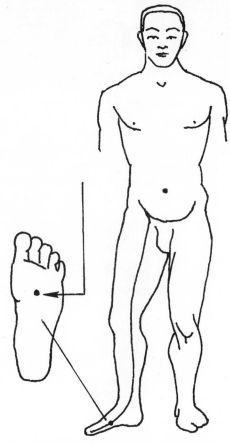

Figure 4-12. Bubbling Well Cavity (Yongquan)

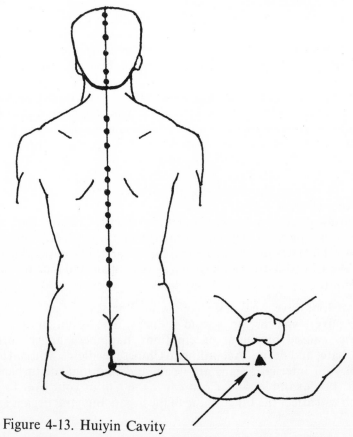

Figure 4-13. Huiyin Cavity

only thing affected—strong emotions also cause Chi to accumulate in your head. When you turn your head from side to side you loosen up the muscles, blood vessels, and Chi channels in your neck, and allow the Chi in your head to smooth out. Additionally, since you are also training your feelings and Shen to be centered and neutral, you will be able to avoid excessive or extreme emotions and their negative effects. In the form you turn your head to look behind you, as if you were looking at all the negative things which you have left behind. It is important to really look to the rear, so that the Chi keeps moving. If you merely turn your head, the Chi will stagnate in your neck. Practicing this piece regularly will regulate the Chi in your organs and head, repairing the damage caused by strong emotions, and helping you to avoid all illnesses.

The poem also implies that this piece can cure old injuries. When you practice, you use your mind to lead the Chi from your Dan Tien to the Bubbling Well cavities, which smooths out the Chi circulation in your lower body. When you turn your head while holding your hands in the different positions, you slightly stretch different parts of the inside of your body and regulate the Chi flow there. This will help to cure old internal injuries and bruises that cannot be easily reached by other methods of treatment.

Fifth Piece:
Sway the head and swing the tail to get rid of the heart fire; (when) heart fire (is) strong, (use) the metal lung to subdue. Hands press the knee caps, repeatedly sway and swing. Blood flows smoothly, many good benefits. (If) the muscles/tendons are cramped, legs sore, (and) body numb, repeatedly extend and press heavily, do not waste time (hesitate).

搖頭擺尾去心火，心火旺盛肺金克。
手按膝蓋多搖擺，血液暢流好處多。
筋攣腿酸身麻木，重抻重壓莫蹉跎。

Practice: Step your right leg one step to the right and squat down in a horse stance. Place your hands on top of your knees, with the thumbs on the outside of the thighs (Figure 4-14). Your Chi is sunk to the bottom of your feet, and your Yi is on the two Bubbling Well cavities. Shift your weight to your left leg and press down heavily with your hand, and line up ("extend") your head, spine, and right leg (Figure 4-15). Stay in this position for about 3 seconds, then return to the original position, and then repeat the same thing on the other side. Turn 12 times in each direction for a total of 24 repetitions.

Discussion: Fire (excessive Chi) in the Middle Dan Tien at the solar plexus can be caused by improper food, breathing unhealthy air, or lack of sleep. This frequently causes heartburn. For this reason it is called Hsin For (heart fire). When excessive Chi accumulates and stagnates in your Middle Dan Tien or heart, the best course of action is to move this fire to the lungs where you can regulate it and put it out with smooth breathing. According to the five element theory (Table 4-1), fire can destroy metal, but metal can also absorb the heat and control fire (Figure 4-16). The lungs belong to the element metal, and the heart belongs to the element fire, and so it is said that the metal lungs can subdue the heart fire. When you hold your hands on your knees with the thumbs to the rear you are expanding your chest, and when you move your body from side to side, you are loosening up the lungs and therefore taking in the excess Chi from

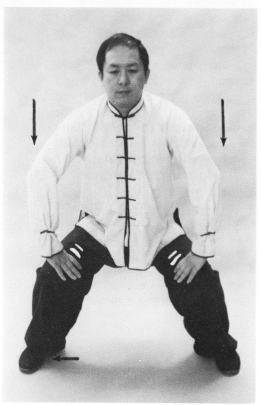

Figure 4-14.

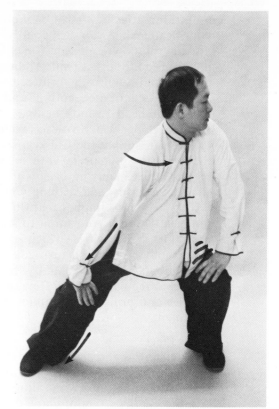

Figure 4-15

	WOOD 木	FIRE 火	EARTH 土	METAL 金	WATER 水
Direction	East	South	Center	West	North
Season	Spring	Summer	Long Summer	Autumn	Winter
Climatic Condition	Wind	Summer Heat	Dampness	Dryness	Cold
Process	Birth	Growth	Transformation	Harvest	Storage
Color	Green	Red	Yellow	White	Black
Taste	Sour	Bitter	Sweet	Pungent	Salty
Smell	Goatish	Burning	Fragrant	Rank	Rotten
Yin Organ	Liver	Heart	Spleen	Lungs	Kidneys
Yang Organ	Gall Bladder	Small Intestine	Stomach	Large Intestine	Bladder
Opening	Eyes	Tongue	Mouth	Nose	Ears
Tissue	Sinews	Blood Vessels	Flesh	Skin/Hair	Bones
Emotion	Anger	Happiness	Pensiveness	Sadness	Fear
Human Sound	Shout	Laughter	Song	Weeping	Groan

Table 4-1. Table of Correspondences associated with the Five Elements

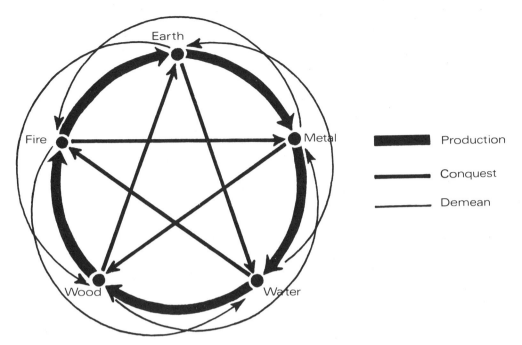

Figure 4-16. Relationship the of Five Elements

the Middle Dan Tien, and consequently putting out the fire. As you are doing this, you are also increasing the blood circulation, which will take care of any numbness or soreness in the legs.

Make sure that when you lean to each side you don't drop your head. Keep your head, neck, and spine in a line. When you "press heavily" on one knee, you compress the lung on that side and relax and open the lung on the other side. This works the two lungs like bellows.

Sixth Piece:
Two hands hold the feet to strengthen the kidneys and waist; (when the) kidneys and waist are strong the entire body (is) strong. Bend the waist and hold the feet. (It is the) most effective way to strengthen the muscles/tendons and bones. One down one up, the life force greatly increases. (It is) the best way to prevent colds.

雙手攀足固腎腰，腎腰充實整體牢。
腎身彎腰手攀足，强筋壯骨有功效。
一落一起活力大，防止感冒更為佳。

Practice: Move your left leg back so that your feet are shoulder distance apart. Press both palms down slightly beside your waist (Figure 4-17), then move your hands up in front of your chest (Figure 4-18) and finally above your head with the palms facing up (Figure 4-19). The form looks as if you were holding or lifting something above your head. Your mind is on your Mingmen cavity in the Kidney area. Stay there for 3 seconds, then bend forward with the arms extended and hold your feet (Figure 4-20). Pull your hands up slightly so that you are putting a gentle stress on your whole body. While holding your feet your mind is on the Bubbling Well cavity. Stay there for 3 seconds. Repeat the entire process 16 times.

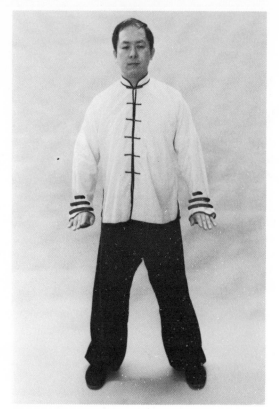

Figure 4-17.

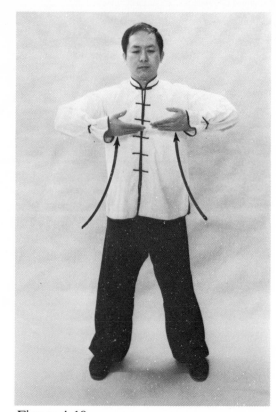

Figure 4-18.

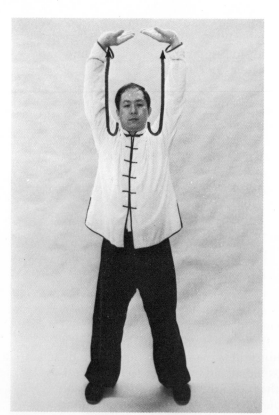

Figure 4-19.

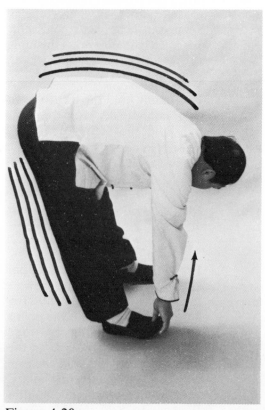

Figure 4-20

Discussion: The kidneys, which are beneath the two major back muscles, are the residence of Original Jieng (Yuan Jieng). When the kidneys are healthy and strong, your Original Jieng is retained and strengthened. Only when your kidneys are strong will they be able to generate Original Chi (Yuan Chi) and enliven your body. When you bend forward and use your hands to hold your feet, you are tensing the back muscles and restricting the flow of Chi in the area of the kidneys. When you release this pressure, the Chi flow will resume, removing any Chi stagnation. This exercise is an excellent way to massage the kidneys and increase the flow of Chi there, as well as in the back muscles and the spine itself. When the kidneys are strong, the Original Chi will be strong. When Original Chi is full and strong, your body will be able to generate a strong shield of Guardian Chi to protect you from the cold.

When you are bent over you are lightly stressing your whole body, and in particular you are stimulating your kidneys. When you straighten up and extend your arms, your mind is thinking of stretching out to your hands and feet. This action of the mind and body leads the Chi out to all your tendons. When you are bent over, part of your attention (and part of the Chi from your kidneys) is drawn to your sacrum. The Chi will enter the spine through the holes in the sacrum, and when you stand up it will pass through the spine. Eventually the Chi will move through and vitalize your whole skeleton.

Seventh Piece:
Screw the fist with fiery eyes to increase Chi Li; body and mind healthy, the spirit of vitality comfortable. Ride the horse and squat down, straightening the chest. Hold the fist or strike with palm, using more force. Left and right, two hands grasp in turn. Grasp, hold, fiery eyes, use Li Chi.

攢拳怒目增氣力，身心健康精神爽。
騎馬蹲襠胸挺直，握拳擊掌多用力。
左右兩手循環抓，抓握怒目用力氣。

Practice: This piece is very similar to the second piece. Step your right foot to the side and squat down in a horse stance, holding your body erect and your fists beside your waist (Figure 4-21). Tighten both fists, and extend one arm to the side in a twisting punch motion ("Screw the fist")(Figure 4-22). Your other hand stays beside your waist in a tight fist. The hand that is out can be either a fist or an open palm. After you finish the extending movement, loosen both hands and bring the extended hand back to your waist to the starting position. Then tighten both hands and repeat to the other side. When you make the punching motion, glare fiercely at an imaginary opponent. Do 8 to either side, for a total of 16.

Discussion: This piece trains you to raise your spirit of vitality. When your spirit is raised, you strengthen the Chi flow and also increase your muscular strength (Li). Muscular strength which is reinforced by Chi is called Chi Li or Li Chi. As you raise your Shen (spirit) and increase your Chi Li, the Chi will fill your body all the way out to the skin. In the other exercises you have been focusing your attention and concentrating your Chi. It is important to now do this piece, because it clears out any stagnant Chi and leads it to the skin. Concentrating your Yi is the key to success. If you have a very strong mental image of punching someone very

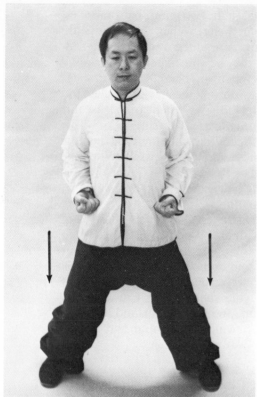
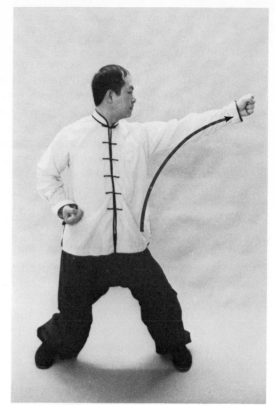

Figure 4-21.   Figure 4-22.

hard, your Yi will lead your Chi out to the ends of your arms and legs to make the punch powerful.

Eighth Piece:
Seven disorders and hundreds of illnesses disappear and are left behind your back; hundreds of illnesses are caused because the body is weak. The feet up, achievement is hard to describe by pen. The head up and press down to reach to the end of the toes. Hold the waist, and hold the chest, up and down movements. (It is) effective in getting rid of sickness and eliminating disasters (illness).

背後七顛百病消 ， 百病皆因體弱招·
足顛功能筆難描 ， 頭頂震到腳趾稍·
招腰捧胸上下顛 ， 祛病消災有攻効·

Practice: There are three parts to this exercise. First, drop both hands down naturally beside your body. Stand still and keep your mind calm. Raise up on your toes and stay as high as you can for 3 seconds, and then lower your feet to the floor (Figure 4-23). Repeat 24 times. Next, place your hands on your waist, and again raise yourself up on your toes for 3 seconds, and then let yourself down. Do this also 24 times (Figure 4-24). Finally, hold your hands in front of your chest and again raise yourself 24 times (Figure 4-25). The different hand positions serve different Chi circulation functions. After you finish this piece, stand still, keep your mind calm, and breathe smoothly and regularly for about 3 minutes.

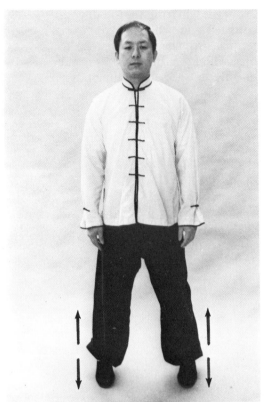

Figure 4-23.

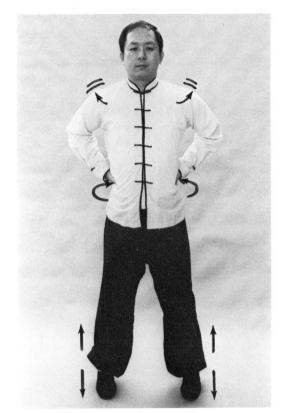

Figure 4-24.

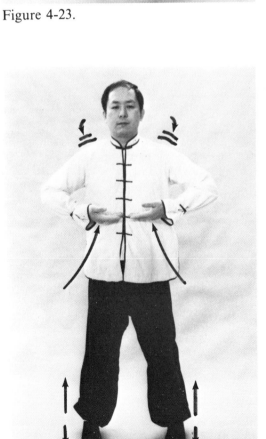

Figure 4-25

Discussion: This piece is used to smooth out the Chi from the top of your head to the bottom of your feet. When you raise yourself up on your toes, you are stimulating six of the Chi channels, which are connected to internal organs. The three hand positions, which are the same as in the fourth piece, help to regulate the Chi in different parts of your body.

CHAPTER 5
CONCLUSION

As mentioned in Chapter 1, Chinese Chi Kung has a number of different styles, or schools, which come from different sources. One style, which was developed by scholars and is now practiced by the general populace, is devoted to maintaining health. The second style was developed by Chinese doctors and concentrates on healing. The third style was developed in the Buddhist and Taoist religions to help the devotees reach the goal of immortality. This style seeks not only to improve and maintain health, but also to lengthen life.

Once you become familiar with the Eight Pieces of Brocade, you will find that it is a very simple but effective way to maintain your health. You may also notice that, unlike the sets developed by doctors and monks, breath coordination is not essential in most of the pieces. The Eight Pieces follow a few simple principles, but they will lead the interested practitioner down the right path to discover what Chi is all about, and will also improve his health.

I hope this simple set of Chi Kung practice will help you to have a healthy life, and encourage you to get involved in further Chi Kung study and research. If you have obtained benefit from this set, please introduce it to your friends and help them to improve their health.

APPENDIX

TRANSLATION OF CHINESE TRMS

About the Author

八段錦 Ba Duann Gin
楊俊敏 Yang, Jwing-Ming
外丹 Wai Dan
氣功 Chi Kung
台灣 Taiwan
功夫/武術 Kung Fu/Wushu
少林 Shaolin
白鶴 Pai Huo
曾金灶 Cheng Gin-Gsao
太極拳 Tai Chi Chuan
高濤 Kao Tao
小週天 Shao Jou Tian
淡江學院 Tamkang College
台北縣 Taipei Hsien
長拳 Chang Chuan
李茂清 Li Mao-Ching
陳威仲 Wilson Chen
張詳三 Chang Shyang-Shan

Foreword and Preface

岳飛宗 Yeuh Fei
南朝 Southern Sung
梁朝 Liang dynasty
忍 Zen

Chapter 1

天氣 Tian Chi
地氣 Di Chi
人氣 Zen Chi
易經 I Ching
三才 San Chai
地理師 Di Li Shy
風水師 Feng Shui Shy
算命師 Suann Ming Shy
漢朝 Han dynasty
梁朝 Liang dynasty
清朝 Ching dynasty
天時 Tian Shyr
人事 Zen Shih
道 Tao
八卦 Ba Kua
氣化論 Chi Far Lun

商 Shang
砭石 Bian Shih
周 Jou
老子 Lao Tzu
李耳 Li Erh
道德經 Tao Te Ching
史紀 Shih Gi
莊子 Chuang Tzu
難經 Nan Ching
扁鵲 Bian Chiueh
金匱要略 Gin Guey Yao Liueh
張仲景 Chang Chung-Gieh
周易參同契 Jou I Chan Ton Chi
魏伯陽 Wei Bo-Yang
禪 Chan
張道陵 Chang Tao-Ling
道教 Tao Jiaw
華陀 Huo Tor
君倩 Juan Gin
五禽戲 Wu Chin Si
葛洪 Gar Hung
抱朴子 Bao Poh Tzu
陶弘景 Tao Hung-Gin
養性延命錄 Yang Shenn Yen Ming Lu
達磨 Da Mo
易筋經 Yi Gin Ching
洗髓經 Shii Soei Ching
隋 Sui
唐 Tang
巢元方 Chow Yun-Fan
諸病源候論 Chu Bin Yun Hou Lun
千金方 Chen Gin Fan
孫思邈 Sun Ssu-Mao
外台秘要 Wai Tai Mi Yao
元 Yuan
養生訣 Yang Shenn Gieh
張安道 Chang An-Tao
儒門視事 Zu Men Shih Shih
張子和 Chang Tzu-Huo
蘭室秘藏 Lan Shih Mi Chan
李果 Li Gou
格致餘論 Ge Tzi Yu Lun
朱丹溪 Chu Dan-Si

張三丰	Chang San-Feng
內丹	Nei Dan
王唯一	Wang Wei-Yi
銅人俞穴鍼灸圖	Torng Ren Yu Hsieh Jen Jeou Twu
仁宗	Ren Tsung
形意功	Hsing Yi
虎步功	Fu Bu Kung
十二叉	Shih Er Chuang
叫化功	Giaou Far Kung
保身秘要	Bao Shenn Mi Yao
曹元白	Tso Yun-Bai
養生膚語	Yang Shenn Huo Yu
陳繼儒	Chen Gi-Zu
精	Jieng
神	Shen
醫方集介庵	Yi Fan Gi Gieh
汪汎庵	Wong Fan-Yen
內功圖説	Nei Kung Twu Shwo
王祖源	Wang Tzu-Yun
火龍功	For Long Kung
太陽掌	Tai Yang Style
八卦掌	Ba Kua Chang
董海川	Tung Hai-Chuan
湯陰縣	Tang Yin Hsien
河南	Henan
鵬	perng
孫子兵法	Suen Tzu Bin Far
孫子	Suen Tzu
周侗	Jou Ton
少林寺	Shaolin Temple
金	Gin
岳家軍	Yeuh Jar Chun
兀朮	Wuh Jwu
拐子馬	Kua Tzu Ma
藤	Tern
藤牌單	Tern Pai Chun
奈檜	Chin Kua
金牌	Gin Pie
何鑄	Ho Juh
精忠報國	Ginn Chung Pau Kuo
岳雲	Yeuh Yun
張憲	Chang Shien
孝宗	Xiao Zong
杭州	Hangzhou
岳武穆	Yeuh Wu Mu
陽	Yang
陰	Yin
陰氣	Ying Chi
營衞氣	Wei Chi
葉明	Yeh Ming
經	Gin
絡	Lou
丹田	Dan Tien
任脈	Ren Mei
督脈	Du Mei

會陰	Huiyin
衝脈	Chong Mei

Chapter 2

調身	Tyau Shenn
調心	Tyau Hsin
調息	Tyau Shyi
調神	Tyau Shen
三寶	San Bao
三元	San Yuan
精子	Jieng Tzu
意	Yi
還精補腦	Huan Jieng Bu Nao
先天氣	Shian Tian Chi
身心衡	Shenn Hsin Pyng Herng
心息相依庵	Hsin Shyi Shiang Yi
李清庵	Li, Ching-Yen
廣成子	Kuan Chen Tzu
唱道真言	Chain Tao Jing Yen Tao
黃庭經	Huang Ting Ching
伍真人	Wu Jen Zen
靈源大道歌	Ling Yuan Da Tao Gar
靜	Jing
細	Shih
深	Shenn
長	Charng
悠	Iou
勻	Yun
緩	Hoan
綿	Mian
內視功夫	Nei Shyh Kung Fu
意守丹田	Yi Shoou Dan Tien
火起	Chii For
以意引氣	Yii Yi Yiin Chi
意氣	Yi-Chi

Chapter 3

閉目靜坐	Bih Muh Jing Tzuoh
上丹田	Shang Dan Tien
中丹田	Jong Dan Tien
下丹田	Shiah Dan Tien
生田神崙	Jiuh Jieng Huey Shen
聚手抱	Shoou Baw Kuen Luen
扣玉	Kow Jyi Yuh Jeen
鳴天鼓	Ming Tian Guu
轉頭頻頻	Joan Tour Pyn Pyn
微擺天柱	Wei Bae Tian Juh
天靈蓋	Tian Ling Gay
臍輪	Chyi Luen
推摩腎俞	Tuei Mo Shenn Yu
手摩精門	Shoou Mo Jieng Men
元精	Yuan Jieng
手轉雙輪	Shoou Joan Shuang Luen
左右轆轤	Tzuoo Yow Luh Lu

-69-